D0396893

EASTMAN'S
EXPECTANT MOTHERHOOD

EASTMAN'S EXPECTANT MOTHERHOOD

by

KEITH P. RUSSELL

M.D., F.A.C.O.G., F.A.C.S.

and

JENNIFER R. NIEBYL

M.D., F.A.C.O.G.

Eighth Edition

Little, Brown and Company

Boston   Toronto   London

EIGHTH EDITION

The photograph on the opposite page is from
the Johns Hopkins University portrait of Dr. Eastman.

Drawings by Jim Chiros on pages 9, 14, 19, 29, 31, 42,
167, 168, 170, 194, 196

Library of Congress Cataloging-in-Publication Data

Eastman, Nicholson Joseph, 1895–
[Expectant motherhood]
Eastman's expectant motherhood / by Keith P. Russell and Jennifer
R. Niebyl — 8th ed., rev.
p.   cm.
Includes index.
ISBN 0-316-76304-7
1. Pregnancy — Popular works.   2. Childbirth — Popular works.
3. Obstetrics — Popular works.   I. Russell, Keith P.   II. Niebyl,
Jennifer R.   III. Title
RG525.E2   1989
618.2 — dc19   89-2789
                                                                            CIP

10 9 8 7 6 5 4 3 2

BP

*Published simultaneously in Canada
by Little, Brown & Company (Canada) Limited*

PRINTED IN THE UNITED STATES OF AMERICA

NICHOLSON J. EASTMAN, M.D.

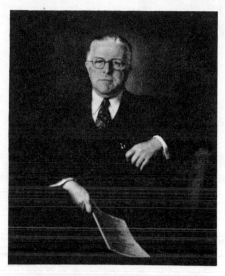

Nicholson J. Eastman, M.D., author of the first four editions of this book and coauthor of the Fifth Edition, died in September 1973. Dr. Eastman was Professor of Obstetrics at Johns Hopkins University and Obstetrician-in-Chief of the Johns Hopkins Hospital, positions that he held for twenty-five years before his retirement. He had also been president of the American College of Obstetricians and Gynecologists, and of the American Association of Obstetricians and Gynecologists. Dr. Eastman originally conceived and wrote this book as a guide for the expectant mother and an adjunct to the physician in her care. The original text and updated revisions have served to improve the understanding and application of sound obstetrical advice for many thousands of mothers and their families over nearly four decades.

The present edition is published in the earnest desire to carry on the high ideals and traditional teachings of Dr. Eastman. He was perhaps the most outstanding teacher-obstetrician of his time, and it is with a deep sense of honor and humility that the present writers succeed him as authors of the Eighth Edition of *Eastman's Expectant Motherhood*.

KEITH P. RUSSELL, M.D.
JENNIFER R. NIEBYL, M.D.

PREFACE TO THE EIGHTH EDITION

Pregnancy should be a healthy, happy time. Childbearing is a natural process, the supreme physical function of womanhood, and no other event confers such deep, abiding contentment. As a rule, most of pregnancy is associated with an increased sense of vitality and well-being. Many of the discomforts, which only a few decades ago were regarded as invariable accompaniments of pregnancy and labor, have been tracked to their source and are now amenable to simple preventive measures; even that old bugbear of childbirth, the pain of labor, can be so managed that the majority of American mothers today experience a minimum of discomfort. Meanwhile, modern methods of care have so surrounded the whole process with multiple safeguards that the likelihood of a serious complication developing is exceedingly remote.

Yes, pregnancy should be a healthy, happy time. But health and happiness in pregnancy are dependent in large measure upon proper guidance by a competent physician, with a team of nurses, technicians, and allied health personnel. There is no substitute for such care, based on the physician's acquaintance with the expectant mother and her individual situation. Your doctor, accordingly, should be your chief guide.

What, then, is the reason for a volume such as this? In the first place, it is common knowledge that women of today often need more information about prenatal care and labor than the physician has time to give them. In the second place, verbal precepts may sometimes be forgotten; and since the recommendations set forth in this book represent accepted principles of prenatal care, it is hoped that it may serve as a sort of stenographic recapitulation of the doctor's main communications, which may be reviewed leisurely at home. Finally, from the viewpoint of both patient and doctor, it is hoped that many of the questions that almost every expectant mother asks will be answered here, so that her visits to the physician may be devoted more largely to the particular circumstances of her individual case.

The obstetrical art advances, and during the six years that have elapsed since the Seventh Edition of *Expectant Motherhood* appeared, various improvements in maternity care have made childbearing an even safer, more comfortable, and happier experience than it was just a short time ago. Having a baby today, provided that you are in the hands of a competent doctor, is a much safer undertaking than a long automobile trip. And as for comfort in labor, numerous effective methods of care at this time await you. Moreover, doctors and nurses everywhere are developing a broader appreciation of the many problems that expectant mothers face, with the result that individual questions are answered with increasing understanding and insight.

The meticulous attention plus great technological advances that are available to today's expectant mother, including those in labor, have made increasing demands on the schedules of doctors and nurses alike. Consequently they often find their time somewhat curtailed for informing the expectant mother as to the many *routine* details of prenatal hygiene that she should know. The reception accorded the first seven editions of *Expectant Motherhood,* as well as innumerable letters from doctors and patients, has encouraged us to believe that this book serves a useful purpose by providing this information in simple, practical form. It is likewise gratifying to be told that it has saved a certain amount of time for physicians the country over by sparing them countless questions in the office and many telephone calls both day and night.

This updated Eighth Edition of *Expectant Motherhood* incorporates the principal advances made in maternity care over recent years to the end that this small volume may continue to serve as a thoroughly modern guidebook for expectant mothers.

KEITH P. RUSSELL, M.D.
JENNIFER R. NIEBYL, M.D.

CONTENTS

xi

Contents

Contents

xiii

Contents

ILLUSTRATIONS

Illustrations

EASTMAN'S
EXPECTANT MOTHERHOOD

1

SIGNS AND SYMPTOMS
OF PREGNANCY

I n ancient Rome it was customary after marriage for a
young woman to wear around her neck a snug-fitting
band of some rigid material such as gold, silver, or brass.
These bandeaux were often exquisitely wrought, but their
main purpose was not ornamental but diagnostic; when
pregnancy supervened, the bandeau would become un-
comfortably tight. Its removal, accordingly, carried an obvious implication and was the occasion of great rejoicing
in the household, for it meant that the young woman had
set forth on the Great Adventure — the creation of a new
life.

Although many centuries have passed since the time of
the Roman bandeau, the first visit of the modern expectant
mother to her doctor is usually prompted by the same
query: "Am I really pregnant?" Oddly enough, this is the
one question which the physician may not be able to answer with certainty, judging by physical examination
alone. There is rarely clear-cut physical evidence of pregnancy before at least two menstrual periods have been
missed. New sensitive pregnancy tests are helpful this
early in pregnancy.

Biochemical and Immunological Tests

In recent years, tests that make use of an immunological reaction to pregnancy hormones in the blood or urine have become widely used. These tests have the advantages of not requiring laboratory animals and of ease and quickness in obtaining results. Most results are available within a few minutes to an hour or two, depending on the method used. It is better that the urine for such tests be concentrated (no fluids for a number of hours before taking the specimen) and that it be fairly recently obtained. These immunological tests have an accuracy approaching 98 percent.

Over-the-counter urine pregnancy tests are usually positive from one to seven days after the first missed period. Sensitive blood tests, usually reserved for special circumstances, can determine the presence of pregnancy as early as a week after conception (a week before a period is missed). Ultrasound methods are useful when the diagnosis of pregnancy remains doubtful or when certain complications occur. Sonographic studies (called sonograms or echograms) can visualize the developing embryonic sac in early stages of pregnancy, and after a few weeks can also visualize the fetal heart action, thus confirming the pregnancy. This method poses no threat to the developing embryo, as it does not utilize X rays.

The Expectant Mother's Observations

Cessation of Menstruation
In a healthy, sexually active woman who has previously menstruated regularly, cessation of menstruation suggests

strongly that impregnation has occurred. Not until the date of the expected period has been passed by ten days or more, however, can any reliance be put on this symptom. There is scarcely a woman who menstruates exactly every twenty-eight or thirty days. Studies have shown that the majority of women (almost 60 percent) experience variations in the length of their individual cycles that exceed five days; differences in the same woman of even ten days are not uncommon and occur without explanation and without apparent detriment to health. When, however, the expected period has been passed by more than ten days, under the circumstances mentioned, the likelihood of pregnancy is good. When the second period is also missed, the probability naturally becomes stronger.

Although cessation of menstruation is the earliest and one of the most important symptoms of pregnancy, it should be noted that pregnancy may occur without prior menstruation, and that bleeding may occasionally continue after conception. For instance, among girls who become pregnant at a very early age, pregnancy frequently occurs before menstrual regularity has become established; nursing mothers, who usually do not menstruate during the period of lactation, often conceive at this time; more rarely, women who think they have passed the menopause are startled to find themselves pregnant. Conversely, it is not uncommon for a woman to have one or two "periods" after conception, but usually these are brief in duration and scant in amount. In such cases the first period ordinarily lasts two days instead of the usual five and the next only a few hours. However, *vaginal bleeding at any time during pregnancy should be regarded as abnormal and reported to the physician at once.*

Absence of menstruation (amenorrhea) may result from

a number of conditions other than pregnancy. Change of climate, weight gain or loss, certain chronic diseases such as anemia, and sometimes emotional strains and anxiety such as concern about an unplanned pregnancy — all may suppress the menstrual flow. In addition, nutritional deficiencies caused by excessively restricted, low-protein diets are a common cause of loss of menstruation.

Breast Changes

Slight, temporary enlargement of the breasts, causing sensations of weight and fullness, are noted by most women prior to their menstrual periods. The earliest breast symptoms of pregnancy are merely exaggerations of these changes. Thus, the breasts become larger, firmer, and more tender; a sensation of stretching fullness accompanied by tingling both in the breasts and in the nipples often develops; and in many instances a feeling of throbbing is also experienced. As time goes on, the nipple and the elevated pigmented area immediately around it — the areola — become darker in color. The areola tends to become puffy, and its diameter, which in nonpregnant women rarely exceeds an inch and a half, gradually widens to two or even three inches. Embedded in this areola are tiny milk glands that take on new growth with the advent of pregnancy and appear as little protuberances, or follicles. These have been called Montgomery's tubercles after a famous Irish obstetrician of the nineteenth century who described them very completely and, in summarizing, created a famous medical pun by saying "They are, in fact, a constellation of miniature nipples scattered over a milky way." These make sebaceous material which provides natural lubrication for the nipple. The tubercles of Montgomery, which appear about the eighth week of

4

pregnancy, may not be noticed by the patient but constitute one of the changes the doctor will probably look for. It is needless to say that all these alterations are directed ultimately at furnishing milk for the baby, and as early as the fourth month — the time varies somewhat — a little silvery-white, sticky fluid may be expressed from the nipple; this is colostrum, a watery precursor of milk. During the latter part of pregnancy this fluid may be sufficient in quantity to necessitate the wearing of a small pad over the nipples to protect the clothes. At the same time it may dry on the surface of the nipples in small flakes, which are often irritating and tend to make the nipples sore; if this occurs, the nipples should be gently washed with warm water (no soap) as often as is necessary and then thoroughly dried. About the fifth month of pregnancy it is frequently observed that patches of brownish discoloration appear on the normal skin immediately surrounding the areola. This is known as the secondary areola and is a result of pregnancy, provided the woman has never previously nursed an infant. With the increasing growth and activity of the breasts it is not surprising that a richer blood supply is needed, and to this end the blood vessels supplying the area enlarge. As a result the veins beneath the skin of the breast, which previously may have been scarcely visible, now become more prominent and occasionally exhibit intertwining patterns over the whole chest wall.

Frequency of Urination

Irritability of the bladder, with resultant frequency of urination, may be one of the earliest symptoms of pregnancy. It is attributed to the fact that the growing uterus stretches the base of the bladder, so that a sensation results identical with that felt when the bladder wall is stretched with urine. As pregnancy progresses, the uterus rises out of the pelvis and the frequent desire to urinate subsides. Later on, however, the symptom is likely to return, for during the last weeks the head of the baby may press against the bladder and give rise to a similar condition. Although frequency of urination may be somewhat bothersome, both at the beginning and at the end of pregnancy, it should never constitute a reason for reducing the quantity of fluid consumed, which should not fall below six to eight glasses a day. If, late in pregnancy, frequency of urination disturbs sleep, the full amount of fluid should be taken before six in the evening and liquid avoided until morning.

Nausea

About one-third of pregnant women suffer no nausea whatsoever. Another third, during the early part of pregnancy, experience waves of nausea for a few hours in the morning, but this does not proceed to the point of vomiting. In the remaining third the nausea may cause actual vomiting. When this "morning sickness" occurs it usually makes its appearance about two weeks after the first missed menstrual period and subsides ordinarily after the third month. Since this symptom is present in many other conditions, such as ordinary indigestion, it is not in itself evidence of pregnancy.

In summary, then, the earliest symptoms of pregnancy are cessation of menstruation, enlargement of the breasts, frequency of urination, and nausea. Although none of these is absolute proof of pregnancy, cessation of menstruation followed by one or more of the other symptoms is strongly suggestive; if two periods are missed and any of the other symptoms is also present, pregnancy is highly probable. Pregnancy tests are usually positive a week or ten days after the first missed period, and ultrasound can usually reveal the fetal heartbeat within seven weeks after the last menstrual period.

Quickening

Quickening is an old term derived from an idea prevalent many years ago that at some particular moment of pregnancy life is suddenly infused into the infant. At the time this notion was in vogue, the first tangible evidence of intrauterine life lay in the mother's feeling the baby move, and the conclusion was only natural that the infant became alive at the moment these movements were first felt. As is reflected in the Biblical reference to the "quick and the dead," the word *quick* used to mean "alive," and the word *quickening* meant "becoming alive." Hence, we said that when fetal movements were first felt, "quickening," or "coming to life," of the baby had occurred. We now know that the infant is a living organism from the moment of conception, but quickening is still often used in obstetrical circles as a term for what is more generally called "feeling life." As used today, quickening refers only, of course, to the active movements of the child as first perceived by the mother. We now know that there are active fetal movements much earlier, as shown on ultrasound examination, which are imperceptible to the mother.

Quickening is usually felt near the completion of sixteen to twenty weeks of pregnancy as a tremulous fluttering low in the abdomen. These sensations caused by the stirring of the baby may be so faint as to raise some doubt as to their cause; later on, however, they grow stronger and often become so vigorous that many mothers are inclined to wonder if the baby is not destined to become an acrobat.

7

Although quite painless, they may occasionally disturb the mother's sleep during the later weeks.

Many babies who are alive and healthy seem to move about very little in the uterus, but it is unusual for a day to pass without some movement being felt. If a day passes without fetal movement in the last half of pregnancy, or fetal movement decreases significantly, the fetus should be evaluated by electronic monitoring tests, such as non-stress tests (see chapter 11). Inability to feel the baby move does not mean that it is dead or in any way a weakling, but in all probability that it has assumed a position in which its movements are not so readily felt by the mother. More-over, it is a well-established fact that the baby in the uterus sleeps, and it seems likely that the periods of active move-ments and quiescence that the mother notices correspond to the phases of wakefulness and sleep. It might seem that the sensations produced by the baby's movements would be so characteristic as to make this a positive sign of preg-nancy, but it is possible for movements of gas in the intes-tines to be misinterpreted as motions of a baby.

Other Changes

As pregnancy advances, other changes will be noted by the expectant mother. As early as the end of the twelfth week she may be able to feel a soft lump just above the pubic bone. This is the pregnant uterus, which gradually enlarges to reach the navel at about twenty weeks and, as shown in Figure 1, eventually fills the greater part of the abdomen. Pregnancy begins to "show" about the time the growing uterus reaches the navel and thereafter the condi-tion is usually obvious. Attempts to conceal it by the use of tight girdles are dangerous; serious accidents have re-sulted from this practice.

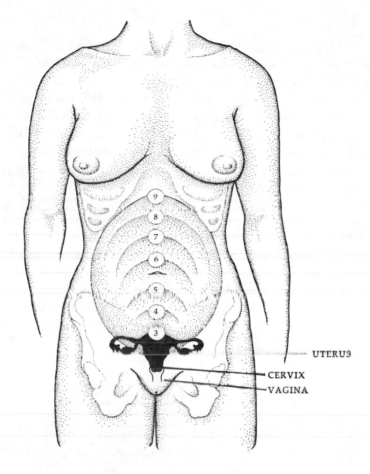

UTERUS

CERVIX
VAGINA

FIGURE 1. Height reached by the uterus at successive months of pregnancy

In current terminology, pregnancy duration is listed by weeks. Thus, term is forty weeks. In the illustration, corresponding weeks of pregnancy are

3 — 12 weeks	6 — 22 weeks
4 — 14 weeks	7 — 28 weeks
5 — 18 weeks	8 — 35 weeks
	9 — 40 weeks

9

During the latter half of pregnancy, pinkish or bluish streaks, resembling little scars or veins, may appear over the lower abdomen. These represent small breaks in the lower layer of the skin, which is less elastic than the upper and gives way in places to the stretching caused by the enlarging uterus. These "stretch marks" are occasionally seen also on the lower parts of the breasts and on the thighs. After the birth of the baby these streaks (striae) remain permanently as silvery-white lines. Most women would like to avoid these tiny blemishes if at all possible, but there is no form of treatment that is certain to prevent them. It may help with the itching that frequently accompanies these marks, however, to massage the skin daily with some lubricant such as olive oil or skin cream.

Another common change in the skin, particularly in brunettes, is the development of a brownish line running from the navel downward to the pubic bone; this fades soon after pregnancy is over and with time almost entirely disappears.

The Physician's Observations

In making a diagnosis of pregnancy the physician will first inquire about the early changes that have just been reviewed and if several of these are present is likely to consider them strong evidence. Since no one of these symptoms is an infallible sign of pregnancy, however, the results of physical examination and laboratory tests will be considered more definitive.

Breast Changes

As a rule the physician begins an examination for the determination of pregnancy by inspection of the breasts, checking up on any alterations noted by the patient such as we have already described (pigmentation, etc.).

Pelvic Examination

Since it is customary (and highly desirable) for a woman to visit her physician as soon as she suspects pregnancy, the doctor is often called upon to make the diagnosis at a stage so early that fetal movements and heart sounds are not yet detectable. The evidence given by the expectant mother and that afforded by the physician's inspection of the breasts must accordingly be supplemented by an examination of the reproductive organs themselves. With the patient completely draped in a sheet and relaxed, the folds of the sheet in the region of the external reproductive organs are separated and the mucous membrane of the vagina inspected. Ordinarily this is pink in color, but early in pregnancy it acquires a dusky bluish tinge. With two fingers of a gloved hand the physician then carries out an internal examination in order to determine whether characteristic changes are present in the uterus itself. If the patient will close her eyes, let all her muscles "go loose," and breathe quietly through her mouth for relaxation, she will not only be helping the physician, but will find that the whole procedure is quite painless. The degree to which the uterus is enlarged, its shape and consistency, are all valuable diagnostic aids that, when considered with the other evidence, usually allow a highly probable diagnosis of pregnancy to be made soon after the second period has been missed.

Fetal Heart Sounds

The abdominal examination comprises palpation of the uterus and, if this has risen well above the pubic bone,

11

listening for the baby's heartbeats. Curiously enough, the knowledge that these heart sounds could be heard came to us more or less by accident. Something over a hundred years ago it so happened that a Swiss physician thought it might be interesting to place his ear over the abdomen of a pregnant woman and try to hear the baby splashing about in the fluid surrounding it. Anticipating splashes, he was amazed to hear faint rhythmic beats that resembled the ticking of a watch under a pillow, and shortly he realized that he was listening — for perhaps the first time in history — to the heartbeats of a baby within the uterus. The rate of the fetal heart is much faster than the usual rate of the maternal heart and ordinarily approximates 140 beats a minute. Under favorable circumstances these sounds become audible about the twentieth week with a stethoscope. With ultrasound techniques the heartbeat can be detected even earlier, usually by the seventh week of pregnancy. Accumulated evidence of other types has usually made the diagnosis already so clear that this final proof is scarcely necessary. Nevertheless, these ticktock messages from within the uterus, proclaiming in unequivocal terms the welfare of the baby, are always reassuring to mother and physician alike.

Fetal Movements

Although, as we have seen, mothers may be mistaken about the sensations they interpret as movements of the baby, the impulse that such a movement conveys to the examining hand of the physician is unmistakable and constitutes a positive sign of pregnancy. These movements, however, are usually not palpable until about twenty weeks.

2

GROWTH AND DEVELOPMENT
OF THE FETUS

I n all nature's wide universe of miracles there is no process more wondrous than the one by which a tiny
speck of tissue, the human conceptus, develops into a cry-
ing seven-pound baby. So miraculous did primitive peoples consider this phenomenon that they ascribed it all to
superhuman intervention, and throughout unremem-
bered ages they worked out various theories as to how the
miracle began.

Now we know that pregnancy comes about in only one
way: from the union of a female cell, the egg (ovum), with
a male cell, the spermatozoon. The eggs (ova) are produced at the rate of one a month by one or the other of the
ovaries, whitish, almond-shaped bodies near the uterus
(see Figure 2). The process by which an ovum and a spermatozoon fuse is usually called fertilization by scientists,
and conception as a general term. After an egg has been
fertilized it naturally requires, like any other egg, a nest or
bed in which to grow. Since a rich bed is essential to the
welfare of the fertilized ovum, let us consider how it is
formed each month and, in passing, consider its relation to
the function of menstruation.

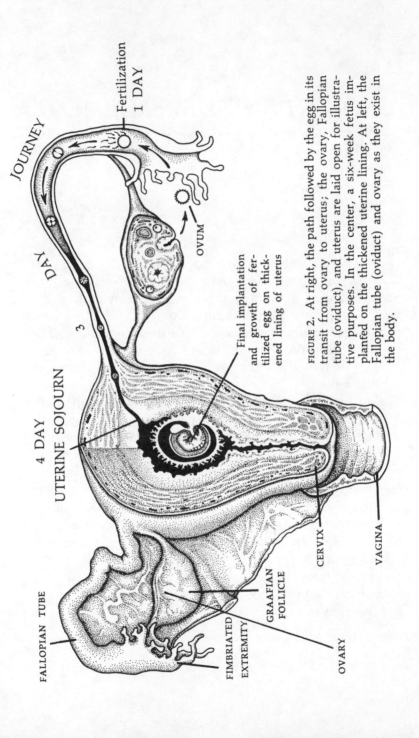

JOURNEY

Fertilization
1 DAY

DAY

3

OVUM

Final implantation
and growth of fer-
tilized egg on thick-
ened lining of uterus

4 DAY
UTERINE SOJOURN

FALLOPIAN TUBE

CERVIX

GRAAFIAN
FOLLICLE

FIMBRIATED
EXTREMITY

OVARY

VAGINA

FIGURE 2. At right, the path followed by the egg in its transit from ovary to uterus; the ovary, Fallopian tube (oviduct), and uterus are laid open for illustrative purposes. In the center, a six-week fetus implanted on the thickened uterine lining. At left, the Fallopian tube (oviduct) and ovary as they exist in the body.

Role of Menstruation in Childbearing

It is well known that the span of years during which childbearing is usually possible corresponds to the period during which menstruation occurs; in general, moreover, a woman who menstruates is able to conceive whereas one who does not is sterile. There is good reason for believing, therefore, that these two phenomena are closely inter-linked, and since no process of nature is meaningless, that menstruation must play some vital and indispensable role in childbearing.

The organ of menstruation, of course, is the uterus (womb), a hollow, pear-shaped, muscular organ that in the nonpregnant state measures about three inches and is joined to the upper end of the vagina in the pelvic cavity. If, day by day, we were privileged to watch the lining membrane of this organ, we should observe some remarkable alterations. Immediately following a menstrual period this membrane is very thin, measuring perhaps a twentieth of an inch in depth. Each day thereafter it becomes a trifle thicker and harbors an increasing content of blood, while its glands become more and more active, secreting a rich nutritive substance that used to be called uterine milk. About a week before the onset of the next expected period this process reaches its height; the lining membrane of the uterus is now the thickness of heavy, downy velvet and has become soft and succulent with blood and glandular secretions. It is at this time and into this luxuriant bed that the egg, if one has been fertilized, sinks.

All these changes have but one purpose: to provide a suitable bed in which the fertilized ovum may rest, secure nourishment, and grow. Now, if an egg is not fertilized, these alterations are unnecessary, and accordingly, through a mechanism that even today is not completely clear, the swollen lining of the uterus disintegrates, the encased blood and glandular secretions escape into the uterine cavity, and, passing through the neck of the uterus, flow out through the vagina, carrying the egg with them. In other words, menstrual bleeding represents the abrupt termination of a process designed to prepare board and lodging, as it were, for a fertilized ovum; its purpose, then, is to clear away the old bed in order that a new and fresh one may be created the next month.

Ovulation and Fertilization

But what happens if the ovum *is* fertilized?

Each month, with punctilious regularity, a blisterlike structure about half an inch in diameter develops on the surface of one or the other ovary. Inside this bubble, almost lost in the fluid surrounding it, lies a tiny speck scarcely visible to the naked eye; a thimble would hold three million of them. This little speck contains within it all that you are heir to; it not only possesses the potentialities for developing into a man or woman, with all the complicated physical organization entailed, but also embodies the mental as well as physical traits of yourself and your forebears: perhaps your own brown eyes or your father's tall stature, possibly your mother's love of music or your grandfather's genius at mathematics. These, and a million other potentialities, are all wrapped up in this little speck, or ovum, so small that it is about one-fourth the size of the period at the end of this sentence.

With the exact periodicity that characterizes so many of nature's works, one blister on one ovary opens at a definite time each month and discharges an ovum, a process known as ovulation. The precise day on which ovulation occurs is a matter of no small importance. For instance, since the ovum can be fertilized only within the twenty-four-hour period after its escape from the ovary, this is the only time at which a woman is really fertile. During the rest of the monthly cycle, theoretically at least, it is impossible for her to conceive. Evidence of various sorts indicates that ovulation usually occurs between the tenth and fourteenth days of the menstrual cycle, counting from the day on which bleeding begins; ordinarily, then, the most fertile time is about a week after the cessation of menstruation. There are, however, many exceptions to this rule, and ovulation may take place at any time between the ninth and eighteenth days of the cycle. The fact that ovulation rarely occurs during the last ten days of a twenty-eight-day cycle has given rise to the birth control doctrine of the "safe period," according to which it is impossible for a child to be conceived after the eighteenth day. Theoretically this claim is altogether sound; practically, many women appear to have conceived during this period, so ovulation may occasionally take place later than theory would have us believe. Ovulation predictors for over-the-counter sale are usually reserved for couples having a problem with conceiving.

After the ovum has been discharged from the ovary it faces a perilous seven-day journey (Figure 2). Its goal is the cavity of the uterus, more than three inches away. The only pathway of approach is the Fallopian tube (oviduct), whose lining is wrinkled unevenly into countless little hills and valleys, and whose passageway at the inner end is no larger than a bristle. The ovum, moreover, has no means of propelling itself through this winding, bumpy tunnel.

Offhand, it would seem an impossible feat; actually, the ovum is not only able to make this journey with apparent ease but has also been known to reach its destination after the most unbelievable meanderings. For instance, if one Fallopian tube has been removed by surgery, the ovum may migrate to the opposite side of the uterus and enter the other tube. This tubal transportation system is made possible, it seems, because of currents in the film of fluid bathing the lining of the Fallopian tube. If we could inspect this lining with a microscope, we should see little hairlike projections (cilia) that wave or beat in such a way as to direct any overlying fluid (as well as any particle it may carry) in the direction of the uterine cavity. Once the ovum has been expelled from the ovary it is drawn by the currents into the funnellike opening of the tube and is thence propelled down the tube by these same currents, as well as by the muscular action of the tubal walls. But it is scarcely a third of the way down the tube when the supreme event happens: it meets a spermatozoon and a new human being is created. As Margaret Shea Gilbert so happily expressed it in her *Biography of the Unborn,* "Life begins for each of us at an unfelt, unknown, and unhonored instant when a minute, wriggling sperm plunges headlong into a mature ovum or egg."

These spermatozoa are in some respects even more remarkable than the ova they fertilize. In appearance they resemble microscopic tadpoles, with oval heads and long, lashing tails about ten times the length of the head. As is shown in Figure 3, they are much smaller than the ovum, their overall length measuring about one-quarter the diameter of the egg, and it has been estimated that the heads of two billion of them could be placed, with room to spare, in the hull of a grain of rice. Yet just as all the physical and

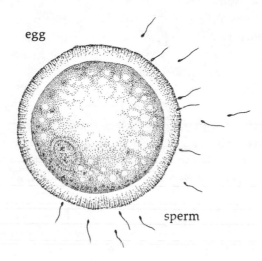

FIGURE 3. Relative sizes of egg (cross-section) and sperm cells

mental traits that you are heir to are contained within the ovum (page 16), so the same kind of inheritance in the male is entirely encapsulated within this infinitely tiny sperm head.

Spermatozoa swim with a quick vibrating motion and have been timed under the microscope at rates as fast as one seventh of an inch a minute. In ascending the uterus and Fallopian tube they must swim against the same currents that waft the ovum downward, but nevertheless they seem able to reach the outer part of the tube within an hour or two. Perhaps the most amazing feature of spermatozoa is their huge number. At each ejaculation, the climax of intercourse in the male, about three hundred million are discharged; if each of these could be united with an ovum, the babies that would thus be started would equal the total number born in the United States during the past one hundred years — all from a single ejaculation. So lavish is nature in her effort to perpetuate the species! Although many million spermatozoa die in the vagina as the result of the acid secretion there, myriads survive, penetrate the neck of the uterus, and swarm upward through the uterine cavity and into the Fallopian tube. There they lie in wait for the ovum.

But they cannot wait long, for they are short-lived, probably living no more than a few days. And, as we have said, the ovum can be fertilized only during the span of a day or so after being discharged from the ovary. By putting these two facts together it will be seen that conception is possible only at the approximate time of ovulation, allowing a day or so before or after for normal variation.

Such an important process as the union of the sperm and ovum — a mechanism upon which all future generations depend — is not left to mere chance but is motivated by a deep-rooted quality all cells of opposite sex exhibit; namely, a violent attraction toward each other. As soon as the ovum comes near the army of spermatozoa, the latter, as if they were tiny bits of steel drawn by a powerful magnet, fly at the ovum. One penetrates, but only one. By what mechanism the countless other sperms are prevented from entering the ovum is not known, but it is well established that as soon as one enters, no others can follow. Now, as if electrified, all the particles making up the ovum (now fused with the sperm) exhibit vigorous agitation, as if they were being rapidly churned about by some unseen force. This agitation becomes more and more violent until it amounts to such an upheaval that the fertilized ovum divides into two cells. This process is repeated again and again, until masses containing sixteen, thirty-two, and sixty-four cells are successively produced, and so on endlessly. Meanwhile this growing aggregation of cells is being carried down the Fallopian tube in the direction of the uterine cavity.

Sex Determination and Heredity

If we could examine an ovum and a sperm head through a high-powered microscope, we should find that each of these cells contains a nucleus, within which a number of dark oval or cylindrical bodies stand out sharply against the surrounding tissues. These are chromosomes, composed of DNA (deoxyribonucleic acid) and protein, which are the carriers of genetic information from the mother and father to the offspring and determine also, as we shall see, the child's sex. We think of a gene as the basic unit of heredity that determines the physical and mental characteristics of an individual. Both genes and chromosomes (carriers of genes) function in pairs. Thus not only the sex of the baby but also all of its physical and mental characteristics are largely predetermined on the basis of genetic probability and chromosomal configuration.

Were we to examine a large number of ova just as the spermatozoa are about to enter them, we should find that each ovum contains exactly twenty-three chromosomes and the sex chromosome in the ovum is called the X chromosome. Likewise, in the sperm we would find twenty-two chromosomes plus a sex chromosome; but here we would note that the sex chromosomes are of two types, one of which is called the X chromosome and the other the Y chromosome. Thanks to the studies of many scientists who have examined these bodies in the utmost detail, we know that when a sperm with an X chromosome fertilizes an ovum, a female infant results, while a sperm with a Y chromosome produces a male. The sex of the future child is, then, ordained the very instant the spermatozoon penetrates the ovum; it depends solely on the type of sex chromosome that particular sperm head happens to possess. Since the number of spermatozoa containing the Y chromosome (boys) is almost the same as the number containing the X chromosome (girls), the sex of the infant is a matter of sheer chance, with the odds about even in the case of full-term children; actually they are slightly in favor of boys by about 106 to 100. In any event, it is the sperm cell of the father that determines the sex of the future baby; the cell of the mother, the ovum, can grow into either a boy or a girl — a fact well worth mentioning to any father who is disappointed by the sex of the child. Although many attempts have been made to influence nature's roulette wheel of sex, so that a child of a desired sex may be had, no consistent success has been met.

If an amniocentesis is performed for prenatal diagnosis, for example for maternal age (see chapter 3), a side benefit is that the chromosome analysis will reveal the infant's sex. Ultrasound examination in late pregnancy may be able to determine the infant's sex with over 90 percent accuracy.

Obviously, when the two sex cells unite, the resulting cell contains forty-six chromosomes, the number present in all the cells of the normal human body except for the sex cells, which, as stated, contain twenty-three.

Embedding of the Fertilized Ovum

The journey of the ovum down the Fallopian tube is believed to require about three days; meanwhile the process of cell multiplication has proceeded to such a degree that the egg, upon entering the uterine cavity, has become a little cluster of cells not unlike a mulberry in conformation. Now the ovum spends a leisurely sojourn of some four days in the uterine cavity, apparently doing nothing. Internally, nevertheless, important changes are taking place. The cells in the center of the egg mass secrete a fluid that pushes the remaining cells to the periphery of the sphere. A specialized portion of the inner layer will develop into the baby. The outer layer is a sort of foraging unit, the trophoblast, which means "feeding" layer; it is the principal function of these cells to secure food for the embryo. It will develop into the placenta, or "afterbirth."

While the ovum is undergoing these changes, the lining of the uterus, it will be recalled, is making preparations for its reception. Considering that ovulation took place on the fourteenth day of the menstrual cycle and that the tubal journey and the uterine sojourn required three and four days respectively, twenty-one days of the cycle will have passed before the ovum has developed its trophoblastic layer of cells. As we have seen, this is just the period when the lining of the uterus has reached its greatest thickness and succulence. In other words, timing has been precisely correct; the bed is prepared and the ovum has so developed that it is now ready to dig into that bed.

The embedding of the ovum is the work of the outer foraging layer of cells, the trophoblast, which possesses the peculiar property of being able to digest or liquefy the tissues with which it comes into contact. In this manner these cells not only burrow into the uterine lining and eat out a nest for the ovum, but also digest the walls of the many small blood vessels they encounter beneath the surface. The mother's bloodstream is thus tapped, and presently the ovum finds itself deeply sunk in the lining bed of the uterus, with tiny pools of blood around it. Sprouting out from the trophoblastic layer, quivering, fingerlike projections now develop and extend into the blood-filled spaces. For the next nine months these fingerlike sprouts serve the fetus as lungs and digestive organs. Through them oxygen, water, and simple foodstuffs such as sugar and calcium pass from mother to child, while in the opposite direction the waste products of the fetus diffuse. At no time, it must be understood, does the blood of the mother mingle directly with that of the fetus; the maternal blood bathes the outside of the trophoblastic projections, the fetal circulation flows within them, and the substances passing from one blood to the other must permeate the walls of these structures.

Bag of Waters and Afterbirth

With the nutritional facilities thus provided, the cells destined to form the baby grow rapidly. At first they all look alike, but soon after embedding, groups of cells here and there assume distinctive characteristics; some develop into bone, some into skin, others into heart, blood vessels, etc. Even before these structures become evident, however, a fluid-filled space develops about the embryo, a space that is lined with a smooth, slippery membrane; this in turn is surrounded by a thicker and stronger membrane. The space is the amniotic cavity, while the membranes and the fluid they contain are often spoken of as the "bag of waters," in which the fetus floats and moves about. The amniotic fluid has a number of important functions. It keeps the fetus at an even temperature, cushions it against possible injury, and provides a medium in which it can move about easily; it is known, furthermore, that the fetus drinks this fluid. At the end of the fourth month of pregnancy the bag of waters has enlarged to the size of a large orange and occupies the entire interior of the uterus.

Meanwhile another important structure has formed, the afterbirth (placenta). This is a fleshy, disclike organ, which late in pregnancy measures about eight inches in diameter and one inch in thickness. It receives its common name from the fact that its birth follows after that of the child; its more scientific name, placenta, derives from the Latin word for cake, which it resembles in shape. The afterbirth, or placenta, is formed by the union of the fingerlike projections of the trophoblast and the lining bed of the uterus into which they sink. An analogous situation is seen when a tree or plant sends down its roots into a bed of earth for nourishment; when the plant is removed a certain amount of the earthy bed clings to the interlocking roots. Similarly a thin layer of the uterine bed clings to the branching projections of trophoblast, and together they make up this organ that supplies food to the baby just as the roots and earth provide nourishment for a plant. The placenta is connected to the fetus by means of the umbilical cord, a gelatinous, coiling structure about twenty inches long. Within it are vessels whose blood carries oxygen and food from placenta to fetus and waste products from fetus to placenta.

Duration of Pregnancy

The length of "term" pregnancy varies greatly; it may range, indeed, between such wide extremes as thirty-seven weeks and forty-two weeks from the last menstrual period and yet be entirely normal in every respect. The average duration, counting from the time of conception, is nine and a half lunar (twenty-eight-day) months; that is, thirty-eight weeks (266 days). Counting from the first day of the last menstrual period, its average length is ten lunar months (forty weeks; 280 days). That these average figures mean very little, however, is shown by the following facts. Scarcely one pregnancy in ten terminates exactly 280 days after the beginning of the last period. Less than one-half terminate within one week of this 280th day. In 10 percent of cases birth occurs a week or more before the theoretical end of pregnancy, and in another 10 percent it takes place more than two weeks later than we would expect from the average figures cited above. Indeed, it would appear that for full development some children require a longer time in the uterus, others a shorter time.

Calculation of the Expected Date of Delivery

In view of the wide variation in the length of pregnancy, it is obviously impossible to predict the expected day of delivery with any degree of precision. The time-honored method, based on the average figures mentioned above, is simple. Count back three calendar months from the first day of the last menstrual period and add seven days. For instance, if the last menstrual period began on June 10, we would count back three months to March 10 and, adding seven days, arrive at the date of March 17. While it may be satisfying to the curiosity to have this date in mind, it must be understood that the likelihood of labor's occurring even within a week of this day is less than 50 percent. There is one chance in ten that it will come at least two weeks later.

And yet, whether pregnancy terminates a week before or two weeks later than the day calculated, the outlook for mother and child is usually just as good as if it had ended at high noon on the due date. Actually, women seldom go "over-term"; in most of these cases it is the above system of calculation and not nature that has erred. For example, ovulation and hence conception may have occurred some days later than usual; this would throw both the beginning and the end of pregnancy just that many days later. If, added to this circumstance, we were dealing with a child who required a slightly longer stay in the uterus for complete development, it would be clear that the apparent delay was quite normal and for the best.

In cases where the last menstrual period is in doubt or ovulation may have occurred late, dating with ultrasound can reduce the frequency of incorrect due dates.

Development of the Baby Month by Month

Most women consider themselves one month pregnant at the time of the first missed menstrual period, two months pregnant at the second missed period, and so on. Since conception does not ordinarily take place until some fourteen days after the onset of menstruation, it is understood that an embryo does not attain the age of one month until about two weeks after the first missed period (assuming a twenty-eight-day cycle). By convention, physicians usually refer to the duration of pregnancy in weeks from the last menstrual period.

End of first lunar month — six weeks (Figure 4). The embryo is about one quarter of an inch long if measured in a straight line from head to tail — for we do have tails at this early stage. The backbone has been laid down but is so bent upon itself that the head almost touches the tip of the tail. At one end of the backbone the head is extremely prominent, representing almost one third of the entire embryo. (Throughout intrauterine life the head is very large in proportion to the body, a relationship that is still present, although to a lesser degree, at birth.) The tube that will form the future heart has been formed and produces a large, rounded bulge on the body wall; even at this early date this structure is pulsating regularly and propelling blood through microscopic arteries. The rudiments of the future digestive tract are also discernible — a long, slender tube leading from the mouth to an expansion in the same tube that will become the stomach; connected with the latter the beginnings of the intestines may be seen. The incipient arms and legs are represented by small budlike nubbins.

End of second lunar month — ten weeks (Figure 4). The embryo now begins to assume human form and hereafter until birth is referred to as a fetus. It has an unmistakably human face and also arms and legs, with fingers, toes, elbows, and knees. During the past four weeks the length of the fetus has quadrupled to about one inch from head to buttocks; the weight is approximately one thirtieth of an ounce. The sex organs become apparent, but it is difficult to distinguish between male and female. It is during the second month that the human tail reaches its greatest development, but by the end of the month it is less promi-

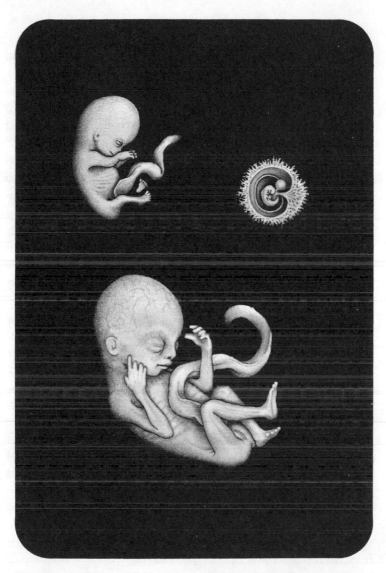

FIGURE 4. Actual size of the fetus at six weeks (shown within the chorionic membrane), ten weeks, and fourteen weeks from the last menstrual period

nent and thereafter undergoes retrogression. The fetal heart can be seen beating on an ultrasound examination.

End of third lunar month — fourteen weeks (Figure 4). The fetus now measures somewhat over three inches in length and weighs an ounce. The sex can now be distinguished by the presence or absence of the uterus. The fingernails and toenails appear as fine membranes. Early in this month buds for all the temporary baby teeth are laid down and sockets for these develop in the jawbone. A rudimentary kidney has developed and secretes small amounts of urine into the bladder, which in all probability escape later into the amniotic fluid. Movements of the fetus are known to occur at this time and can be seen by ultrasound. The fetal heart can now be heard by Doppler ultrasound. The movements are too weak to be felt by the mother.

End of fourth lunar month — eighteen weeks (Figure 5). The fetus from head to toe is now six and a half inches long and about four ounces in weight. A fine downy growth of hair appears on the skin (so-called lanugo hair) and perhaps a few hairs on the scalp. At the end of this period faint movements of the fetus (quickening) may be felt by the mother, but usually these are not experienced until the next month.

End of fifth lunar month — twenty-two weeks. The length of the fetus is approximately ten inches; its weight is about eight ounces. It is at this period that the physician is often able to hear the fetal heart with a stethoscope unaided by Doppler for the first time and that the mother, as we have noted, first feels the baby move. If a fetus is born now it may make a few efforts to breathe, but its lungs are insufficiently developed to cope with conditions outside the uterus and it invariably succumbs within a few hours at most.

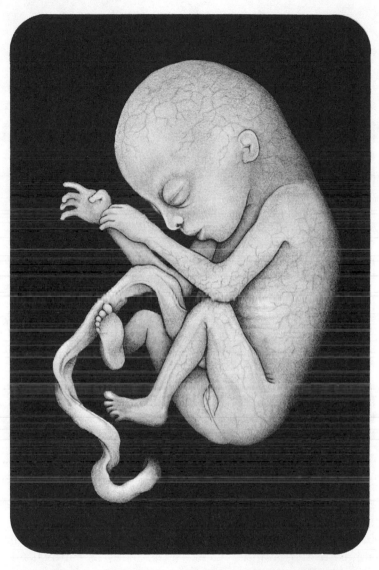

FIGURE 5. Actual size of fetus at eighteen weeks from the last menstrual period

End of sixth lunar month — twenty-six weeks. The length of the fetus is twelve inches and its weight a pound and a half. It now resembles a miniature baby, except that the skin is wrinkled and red, with practically no fat beneath it. At this time, however, the skin begins to develop a protective covering, the vernix caseosa ("cheesy varnish"). This fatty, cheesy substance adheres to the skin of the fetus and at term may be an eighth of an inch thick. Survival at this age is dependent on the availability of neonatal intensive care facilities.

End of seventh lunar month — thirty weeks. The fetus measures about fifteen inches in length and weighs approximately two and a half pounds. If born at this time it has a high chance of survival. There used to be a superstition that infants born at the seventh month would be more likely to survive than those born at the eighth month, a wholly fallacious idea. The fetus born at the eighth month stands a much better chance of survival than one born at the seventh.

End of eighth lunar month — thirty-four weeks. The fetus measures about sixteen and a half inches and weighs some four pounds. With good care, infants born at the end of the eighth month have a great likelihood of survival.

End of ninth lunar month — thirty-eight weeks. For all practical purposes the fetus is now a mature infant, measures some nineteen inches, and weighs around six pounds. As if to improve its appearance before making its debut into the world, the fetus devotes the last two months in the uterus to putting on weight, and during this period gains almost a half-pound a week. Its chances of survival are now about as good as if born at full term.

Middle to end of tenth lunar month. Full term has now been reached, and the fetus weighs on an average about seven pounds if a girl and seven and a half if a boy; its length approximates twenty inches. Its skin is now white or pink and thickly coated with the cheesy vernix. The fine downy hair previously covering its body has largely disappeared. The fingernails are firm and protrude beyond the end of the fingers. The breasts in both boys and girls are often firm and protruding because the same substance that causes the mother's breasts to enlarge during pregnancy passes through the placenta and stimulates development of the fetal breasts. This enlargement subsides within a few days after birth.

Maternal Impressions

No discussion of the growth and development of the baby would be complete without consideration of the old belief that the mental condition of the mother may modify the development of the unborn infant, or, as they used to say, "mark" it. In earlier times many a young woman, for the sake of her unborn child, would struggle to be always cheerful so the child would have a cheerful disposition, or play the piano to ensure a musical gift, or avoid the zoo or circus lest some startled reaction of hers to a strange animal might mark the baby with its likeness.

This belief, like most obstetric superstitions, is of great antiquity: the Biblical story of Jacob and the "speckled and spotted kine" reflects it, while dramatists and novelists from Shakespeare to Dickens have perpetuated the idea in stirring dramas. The facts are these. There is not the slightest nervous connection between mother and child; in other words, there are no possible pathways along which any such impulses, pleasant or otherwise, could travel. The blood of the mother is likewise separate and distinct from that of the child. In addition, all modern experience refutes the belief. Obstetricians of vast experience, as well as maternity hospitals whose annual deliveries run into the thousands, are unanimous in asserting that they have never seen an authentic case.

Finally, as we have seen in the discussion of chromosomes (page 21), your child's mental characteristics are far more deeply rooted than the old legend assumes; they were determined in good measure when your own mother and father, and your partner's, were married. You both, fortunately, have plenty of opportunity to develop an atmosphere and an environment in which your child's capacities (as well as yours and your partner's) can grow and flourish. But whether these talents will lie in the direction of machinery or music or mathematics, or all three, or something else entirely, will not be affected in the slightest by anything you think, see, or hear during pregnancy.

3

VISITS TO THE PHYSICIAN

The Chinese count a person's age not from the day of birth but from the time of conception, a good way of reminding others of what the expectant mother knows — that all this time a living human creature is being nourished who will soon be "nine months old." During this vital formative period the child is in greater need of proper nourishment and suitable environment than at any other stage in life.

The well-being of the baby in this period, as well as in the years to come, naturally depends upon the health of the mother; moreover, her own future well-being is based in substantial degree on her condition during the prenatal months. Accordingly, it is best to place yourself at the earliest possible moment in the hands of a competent physician. Your doctor will have many helpful suggestions about the kinds of food that should be eaten to ensure the growth of a healthy baby, and the routines most conducive to its development, as well as advice regarding details of personal hygiene that can do much to eliminate minor discomforts. These directions about maintaining the highest standards of health will impose no serious deprivations; in fact, the program recommended will prove to be little more than a normal, wholesome life with particular attention to food, proper fluids, elimination, exercise, rest, and sleep — the basic elements we all need to review from time to time to make sure we are looking after ourselves properly.

First Visit to the Physician

The physician first inquires into your past health and that of your parents and the father; the purpose is to ascertain whether there are any past illnesses or hereditary tendencies that might be intensified or aggravated by pregnancy; if there are, precautionary measures are instituted. If there have been previous pregnancies, the doctor reviews these searchingly. Since menstruation is so closely associated with childbearing, questions are asked about the past menstrual history; and in order to fix some approximate date for the expected delivery, the date of the last period is noted.

The greater part of the examination is identical to one that any thorough physician carries out with any patient. As a rule, the first item on the program is for you to be weighed. You will then have a cuff put on your upper arm for a blood pressure reading. These two aspects of the examination (checking your weight and your blood pressure) are almost the only ones that will have to be repeated at all subsequent visits. The latter is of the utmost importance, since a rise in blood pressure is the very earliest sign of a common complication, preeclampsia, formerly called toxemia of pregnancy, which we shall discuss more later. The teeth and throat may then be inspected, and possibly a suggestion to visit a dentist in the near future may be given (see the section on "Teeth," page 87). The physician listens to the chest with a stethoscope to make sure the heart and lungs are normal. Examination of the breasts is important for two reasons: first, in early cases, to obtain confirmatory evidence of the existence of pregnancy, as we have seen in chapter 1; and second, to give advice about nursing. Examination of the abdomen varies with the duration of pregnancy. If your visit is early in pregnancy, as it should be, the doctor will simply make note of the general contour of the abdomen. If you are further along, the size of the uterus is recorded, the position of the baby determined, and its heart sounds listened to. The abdominal examination is usually repeated at subsequent visits, particularly during the later months, because it is naturally important for the doctor to know that the baby is growing and lies in a favorable position.

Labor, the process by which the baby is born, resolves itself largely into the passage of the infant through a bony canal, the pelvis; and it goes without saying that if labor is to proceed smoothly, this canal must be of adequate size. Measurement of the pelvis is therefore performed. It is, however, the inside of the pelvis through which the baby must pass, and one internal examination, to make sure that the internal measurements are ample, is made at some time in the prenatal course. Many physicians carry this out at the first visit, while others prefer a later time. In any event, as we have said, if you relax, the internal examination is not painful and will be over in a few seconds. At the time of the internal examination, a Pap smear is taken to screen for cervical cancer cells.

Finally, as a rule, several tubes of blood are taken from a vein in the arm by means of a fine needle. This "stick" is never pleasant, but the discomfort is momentary, and a careful study of the blood is desirable for several reasons. In the first place, because the fetus and growing uterus consume a great amount of iron, from which hemoglobin (the oxygen-carrying red pigment of our blood) is built, many pregnant women develop anemia; that is, impoverishment of the blood. If the hemoglobin concentration in the blood is low, it is most important for the doctor to know this, since the addition of a little iron to the diet will ordinarily remedy the condition. Another reason for taking a blood sample is to determine the Rh factor, as discussed on pages 48–50. Still another purpose is to rule out the presence of syphilis. Although the vast majority of cases of syphilis are transmitted by sexual relations, a very small number are traceable to other means of exposure. A person may acquire the infection and be quite unaware of its presence, since many years may pass before serious symptoms arise. Nor does the disease apparently affect the well-being of the pregnant woman. Its effect on the unborn child, however, is disastrous. The disease passes to the fetus through the placenta; the fetus usually succumbs and the premature delivery of a dead child follows. If the child is born alive it is very likely to be so feeble that it dies in the first few days or weeks of life. Even if the child survives this period, it still harbors the infection and becomes the victim of various manifestations of the disease later on. Although this picture is very distressing, it is gratifying to know that the treatment of syphilis in the pregnant woman exerts a particularly beneficial effect on the unborn child, and if the treatment is adequate the infant frequently escapes unscathed. During recent years public health officials have shown growing concern about the prevalence of syphilis in the United States and have emphasized the harm it is likely to do to future generations. As a result, most states refuse to grant marriage licenses until both parties are proved by means of one of the standard tests to be free of syphilis. Such a test is also required in pregnancy. In some states prenuptial blood testing for rubella (German measles) immunity is also required, which is otherwise checked in early pregnancy also. A patient can be immunized against rubella after the baby is born, after which contraception is recommended for 3 months.

Patients in high-risk groups, such as those having a history of blood transfusion or intravenous drug abuse, may also be offered testing for hepatitis and HIV, the virus causing AIDS.

While the patient is dressing, the physician arranges for an analysis of the urine. It is the custom of some doctors to ask their patients to bring a morning sample of urine at each visit; others provide arrangements for the patient to furnish a fresh sample in the office lavatory. The urine, like the blood pressure, sometimes shows alterations warning of impending preeclampsia and is examined at each visit. Urine is also checked for infection that is not producing symptoms but may lead to kidney infection later in pregnancy (chapter 8).

Subsequent Visits to the Physician

In the early months of pregnancy, one visit a month to the doctor is ordinarily adequate. During the last half, more frequent examinations are desirable (every two or three weeks), and during the last month every week. At these visits, after asking about your general well-being, the physician measures your blood pressure, analyzes the urine, and records your weight. Some doctors carry out abdominal examinations on each of these occasions, while others do so only during the last two months. As a rule physicians do not charge for these individual visits but include this service (regardless of the number of office visits) in their fee for delivery. This allows you complete freedom to telephone or visit the doctor whenever symptoms warrant it without consideration of expense; at the same time it removes a certain hesitation the physician might have in requesting more frequent visits than usual.

To acquaint you with the hospital and the labor and delivery suites, as well as with some of the procedures you will encounter, many hospitals have tours for expectant parents. These are usually scheduled at regular intervals, or as part of a prepared childbirth class. Your doctor will be glad to arrange for you to attend such a session at the hospital where you plan to have your baby, or, if such tours are not available, make an appointment for you to visit the maternity department individually.

Do not hesitate to bring to your doctor any question that may be bothering you. Above all, as this great event in your life develops, rely on the doctor rather than others for information on any matter concerning your health or well-being, or that of your baby. This advice is not intended to discourage your sharing experiences with friends, or reading, studying, and becoming prepared (childbirth classes) for all aspects of your new circumstances and their eventual outcome. It is intended mainly to help you in regard to any worries and fears arising (as may happen) from dubious advice, old superstitions and taboos, and even tales of woe and disaster that may come your way. If you find yourself in such a position, confide in your doctor as soon as possible. The truth, based on medical facts and combined experience in thousands of maternity cases, should free you from needless concern.

Amniocentesis

Under certain circumstances your doctor may recommend a procedure known as amniocentesis. A common indication is maternal age over thirty-five years, when the incidence of chromosomal abnormalities such as Down syndrome increases. Also if the alpha-fetoprotein value in the blood is abnormal, the test may be offered (p. 47). The test consists of obtaining some of the amniotic fluid (the "bag of water" that surrounds the fetus within the uterus), and performing various examinations on this fluid. The position of the fetus and placenta are first determined by ultrasound examination. The procedure consists of inserting a thin hollow needle through the abdomen and into the uterus, thus entering the amniotic sac (Figure 6). A sample of the fluid is withdrawn, usually about three or four teaspoonfuls, and the needle is then removed. The fluid that has been taken out is readily replaced by the body in a very short time. Most women do not find the procedure painful, except for the slight pinch when local anesthetic is injected into the skin, or when the diagnostic needle is introduced.

The amniotic fluid contains chemicals and hormones that can be analyzed, indicating the welfare of your baby. It also contains cells the baby has shed as it grows. These cells can be grown in tissue culture and analyzed, thus determining the chromosome pattern of the baby. This procedure of tissue culturing usually takes two to three weeks to accomplish. Around the sixteenth week, chromo-

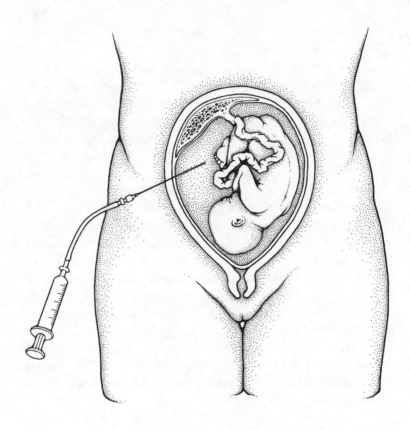

FIGURE 6. Amniocentesis: Amniotic fluid is withdrawn
by needle for testing for certain fetal abnormalities

somal studies of the amniotic cells in the fluid can detect certain genetic disorders in the fetus, such as mongolism (Down syndrome). Later in pregnancy the fluid can be analyzed for information regarding the presence and severity of Rh disease in susceptible infants, or to monitor the development of the fetus. Analysis of the amniotic fluid contents helps to ascertain the stage of maturity of the baby's lungs (L/S ratio), kidneys, and other organs, as well as indicating in some cases if the baby is truly "postmature" or overdue. When a mother requires a "repeat" cesarean section, or planned delivery for medical reasons, amniocentesis is often helpful in setting the date for the delivery.

Examination of the cells shed by the fetus can also be studied to determine the sex of your baby, although the procedure should not be undertaken simply for that purpose since such information is not usually necessary to the management of your pregnancy, and there is a slight risk involved. You will learn soon enough whether you have a boy or a girl! The excitement of anticipation and expectancy is one of the joys of pregnancy many women cherish. Also, the total procedure is often quite expensive, especially if chromosomal studies are performed. You should discuss this and other aspects of the procedure with your doctor.

Because fetal cells may enter the mother's circulation, those few women who are Rh negative should receive immune gamma globulin (Rho-Gam) to prevent Rh sensitization from the procedure. (This type of sensitization is discussed in the next section.)

Occasionally more than one amniocentesis is necessary to obtain the information desired, for example, when the doctor is unable to obtain fluid on the first attempt or when the laboratory is unable to make a proper analysis of the fluid. However, neither of these problems occurs very frequently. Amniocentesis may be repeated also when maturity and related development of your baby is being followed. Amniocentesis is a relatively safe procedure, but there are certain risks, which your doctor can explain. The chance of a miscarriage from the procedure is not great; recent large studies have shown that amniocentesis did not significantly increase the occurrence of miscarriage. (It is important to remember that even after the third month of pregnancy miscarriages can occur spontaneously.)

Amniocentesis can be performed anytime during pregnancy after the fifteenth week. Amniocentesis as early as eleven to twelve weeks is currently being evaluated in some centers. It is usually carried out when there is concern about a possible genetic problem, or when the mother is over thirty-five years old. Later in pregnancy, amniocentesis is done to determine the maturity of the baby (when there may be a question as to the duration of the pregnancy) or to gain information about the condition of the baby. Amniocentesis can be performed either in the hospital or in the doctor's office on an outpatient basis.

Ultrasound (Sonogram) Examinations

Sonography (or ultrasound) is now widely used for a variety of indications. In this procedure sound waves rather than X rays are used to outline the fetus and its various developing structures, to locate the placenta, or to estimate the size and age of the infant while in the uterus.

Sonography may also indicate when twins or other multiple pregnancies are present.

Ultrasound examinations can be used early in pregnancy to determine if in fact the germinal sac is developing, when there may be a question about a possible miscarriage. It is also helpful in diagnosing ectopic (tubal) pregnancy in many cases. Later in pregnancy it will show the development of the fetal skeleton, the heart, and the head. However, if it is done too soon it may give questionable information. Later in pregnancy (near term), it may be used to help diagnose the position of the baby, the size of the infant's head, and the location of the placenta, as mentioned above. It is most frequently used at that time when there is unaccountable bleeding associated with the pregnancy.

It is reassuring to know that the ultrasound examination is painless, quick, and believed to be thoroughly safe. In over twenty years of study by seasoned investigators, there have been no reports of harm to the mother or her developing child by use of this diagnostic technique. Most expectant mothers find the procedure reassuring; frequently, photographs can be taken of the images of the various fetal tissues that are reflected on the TV screen.

There is, of course, an extra fee for these examinations and most doctors recommend them only when there are specific medical indications. Your doctor is in the best position to know when examinations such as sonography and amniocentesis should be done and will advise you about such procedures in greater detail. It is important for you to remember that no procedure is 100 percent accurate, and, as in all laboratory and technical examinations, there is a margin of error or there may be incomplete findings.

Chorionic Villus Sampling

This new procedure allows certain prenatal diagnoses to be made as early as eight to ten weeks, by taking a sample of the chorionic villi, or the tissue destined to become the placenta. In some cases this can be done vaginally, with the patient positioned as if for a pelvic examination. The doctor passes a catheter through the cervix and takes a sample of the villi under ultrasound guidance. If there is distortion of the uterine shape, for example by fibroids, or if the uterus is tipped backward, the villi may be sampled through a needle passed through the abdominal wall.

If an abnormality is detected, the early diagnosis allows earlier and safer pregnancy termination than if the diagnosis is not made until the midtrimester, as with amniocentesis.

Sometimes the results of chorionic villus sampling are difficult to interpret because the placenta may have a slightly different chromosomal arrangement than the fetus, a "mosaic." In about 1 percent of cases of chorionic villus sampling, amniocentesis is required for confirmation.

Alpha-Fetoprotein Testing

A blood test to screen for birth defects is now being widely offered. Alpha-fetoprotein (AFP) is a protein substance made in the fetus which can be detected in the mother's blood. It is higher than normal in cases of certain birth defects such as spina bifida (open spine). It can also be elevated when the fetus is entirely normal, if some of the fetal blood leaks across the placenta into the mother's circulation.

The blood test is usually done at sixteen to eighteen weeks. If the AFP level is high, a repeat value, or reading, may be required. A sonogram to check for twins, error in dates, and obvious abnormalities is also done. If no explanation is found, an amniocentesis is offered to check the level in the amniotic fluid, and a very detailed ultrasound examination is performed to look for birth defects. Sometimes no abnormalities are found, but a very high value may predict a pregnancy complication.

It has recently been recognized that a low value of alphafetoprotein may indicate an increased likelihood of a Down syndrome infant; so amniocentesis may be offered in this situation to mothers even younger than thirty-five years of age.

If the mother elects CVS, alpha-fetoprotein must be sampled later, usually at sixteen weeks, as the fetus only makes minute quantities in the first trimester.

Glucose Screening

Because the hormones of pregnancy increase the need for insulin production by the pancreas, your doctor may test you for diabetes in the last three months of pregnancy, usually around twenty-eight weeks. A standard amount of sugar is given, either in a sweet drink or as a standardized meal, and the blood is drawn one hour later. If the level of blood sugar is normal, no further testing is required. If it is elevated, a full three-hour glucose tolerance test is performed to see if there is any tendency to diabetes.

Pregnancy-induced (gestational) diabetes can usually be treated by attention to a special diet avoiding concentrated sweets.

This is important because untreated gestational diabetes may lead to excessive growth of the baby, as it is exposed to high levels of blood sugar from the mother. This may cause obstetrical difficulties in delivery and put the baby at risk for low blood sugar in the nursery. However, with treatment with a careful diet, these complications can be prevented.

Diagnostic Testing

Jewish women should be screened for the possibility of carrying Tay-Sachs disease. This is a severe neurological disease inevitably ending in death of the child by three or four years of age. The gene occurs once in thirty women in the Jewish population and only once in 300 women in the non-Jewish population. Black women are at risk of sickle cell disease and can be screened for the carrier status.

The Rh Factor

The Rh factor, a substance that most people have in their blood, derives its name from the first two letters of the word *Rhesus;* this factor is always present in the blood of the Rhesus monkey. The Rh factor is present in about 85 percent of Caucasians, 93 percent of Negroes, and 99 percent of Orientals. People with the Rh factor are termed Rh positive; those without it Rh negative.

Once in every several hundred pregnancies, as the result of an extraordinary combination of chance factors, the Rh substance may be responsible for a chain of events that exerts a harmful effect on the fetus. A number of circumstances must be present before this singular action on the fetus can be exerted, as follows: in the first place, the mother must be Rh negative, and as indicated above, there is only about one chance in seven that any member of the white race belongs to this minority group, even less for blacks (about one in fourteen), and still less for Asians (one in a hundred). In the second place, the father of the baby must be Rh positive, and though chances are good that he is in the positive group, he may not be. In the third place, the fetus must be Rh positive, and statistics show that the spermatozoa of about one-fourth of Rh positive men have the potential to produce an Rh negative infant. In the fourth place — and this is the most unlikely circumstance in the lot — the Rh substance from the Rh positive fetus must find its way through the placenta and into the bloodstream of the Rh negative mother and build up antibodies there just as occurs with an Rh positive blood transfusion. Once these antibodies have been developed in the mother, they pass through the placenta into the fetal bloodstream, where they cause varying degrees of damage to the infant's red blood cells. Thus the final factor is that the woman must have had a previous sensitizing pregnancy or blood transfusion to set the chain of events into motion.

From the above facts the following rather comforting conclusions can be drawn. Six out of seven women are Rh positive, with no possibility whatsoever of complications occurring from this source. Furthermore, in first pregnancies, even if the expectant mother is Rh negative, the possibility of trouble developing is practically nil unless she has had a previous blood transfusion with Rh positive blood. But if a woman is Rh negative and has had a previous pregnancy or transfusion, what is her outlook in subsequent pregnancies? The facts are that the vast majority of this group — 90 to 95 percent — go through pregnancy after pregnancy without any suggestion of a complication even if they have not had treatment.

Currently, a method is used that will prevent sensitization to the Rh factor, provided it has not already occurred. This method involves the use of specially prepared serum (gamma globulin), which is given by injection to the Rh negative mother within seventy-two hours after she has delivered an Rh positive infant. This special globulin contains a concentration of Rh antibodies providing protection against foreign Rh positive red cells that may enter the mother's circulation during or after delivery. An injection of this substance provides virtually complete protection by preventing the mother's body from producing her own permanent antibodies.

As some fetal cells may enter the mother's circulation during pregnancy but before delivery, most doctors now recommend giving the Rh immune globulin at about twenty-eight weeks of pregnancy and again after delivery.

The special anti-Rh immune globulin is injected intramuscularly into the nonimmunized Rh negative mother each time she delivers an Rh positive baby, during each pregnancy, after amniocentesis, or after a pregnancy loss. There are no adverse reactions to the injection other than some temporary soreness at the site of injection.

With continued use of this treatment, Rh disease of the newborn is becoming a thing of the past. It should also be pointed out that even if blood disease does arise in the newborn, prompt pediatric care and blood transfusion save 95 percent of the affected live-born infants.

Visits to the Physician

Antenatal Surveillance

Much information can be gained by looking at the baby's heart rate on an electronic fetal monitor before labor. Evaluation of the pattern at rest is called the nonstress test, in which situation accelerations of the fetal heart rate related to fetal movements are checked (see Figure 8, chapter 11). If the baby's heart rate does not accelerate with fetal movements, the stress of contractions may be induced. This can be done by infusing oxytocin to cause uterine contractions, or by stimulating the nipples, which will also result in uterine contractions, just as it does when the baby nurses later. Usually this is done until three contractions are seen in a ten-minute period and the baby's heart rate responce is evaluated.

The baby may also be examined by ultrasound in more detail than just for measurements. In the so called bio physical profile, fetal behaviors such as tone, movements, and breathing, as well as amniotic fluid volume, are noted. All of these tests are used to detect the baby's well-being before it is born.

The tests may be recommended in any situation in which the baby is at risk of not growing well or of needing delivery for distress, such as high blood pressure, diabetes, or being past the due date. These tests reassure the physician of the well-being of the baby before it is born. If they show abnormality they may lead to indicated delivery.

4

NORMAL PSYCHOLOGICAL CHANGES IN PREGNANCY

As we said in the beginning of this book, pregnancy should be a happy, healthy time, representing as it does the supreme physical function of womanhood and the creation of a new life. However, it is also a time of certain emotional reactions that are sometimes difficult for an expectant mother and father to understand. These reactions vary during pregnancy so we will look at them during the three trimesters, or three-month segments, of pregnancy.

First Trimester

Some women feel energetic and look, act, and feel fulfilled even before they know they are pregnant. Others feel tired, frustrated, and depressed. Most expectant mothers alternate between these moods, with the sudden unexplainable shifts of mood contributing to their anxiety. At the outset it should be stated that these reactions are quite normal and common. Very rarely do most pregnant women have true "nervous breakdowns," and it is the experience of many psychiatrists that the occurrence of major emotional disturbances are relatively less common in pregnant women than in their nonpregnant counterparts.

Nonetheless, the psychological impact of a first pregnancy is considerable. It promises major changes in the lives of both parents and, like many major decisions in our lives such as going to college, getting married, or starting a new job, is accompanied by misgivings even after the decision is made. What is mainly required is time for adjustment. Issues at this time will involve letting go of elements of the previous lifestyle — such as certain freedoms, time to oneself, a career perhaps, one income temporarily or longer — and will involve concern for the future, and one's ability to be a good parent, provide a secure home, cope with the demands of a very dependent child, and similar adjustments.

Physically the mother undergoes change during this period too. Hormonal variations take place in the early months of pregnancy, and fatigue is characteristic of this early period, too. Some women will experience "morning sickness," the nausea or actual vomiting that may start around the end of the first month and last a month or two. Bowel irregularity, frequent urination, and vaginal discharge are also commonly encountered, along with swelling and tenderness of the breasts.

When one steps back and looks at all the changes to be dealt with, the sense of emotional vulnerability and the need for adjustment are quite understandable. The important thing to remember when you feel a sense of inadequacy or anxiety, frustration or depression is that these are a normal part of the adjustment process.

Second Trimester

By the fourth month, much of the adjustment discussed above has been accomplished. During this period pregnancy starts to show as the body image changes, and this can be both a source of pride and concern, depending on the mother's attitude. It is also during this period that the baby's movements begin to be felt, so it is an exciting time. The fatigue and nausea of the first months have lessened and that helps too, making this period the more emotionally stable part of a pregnancy for most women. Most women have an increased sense of well-being, and more energy, during this period.

Third Trimester

As the baby increases in size, physical discomfort becomes a feature of this period. The size and weight of the baby affect the mother's balance and posture, requiring more care in movement. Backache is common as the mother tries to compensate for the weight in front of her. Pressure on the bladder and diaphragm make frequent trips to the bathroom and shortness of breath common features at this time as well. The excitement of the first movements of the baby has worn off and its kicking can now be uncomfortable and sometimes irritating. Weight gain is of greater concern during this period than the others. As time goes on, sexual activity and sleep become more awkward or difficult. Fatigue and irritability increase again. The last weeks of pregnancy are often characterized by impatience to deliver and end this period, and concern about how labor will go now that it is close. This latter concern is naturally considerably greater for women pregnant for the first time. This is also the time when expectant mothers will worry about their baby being normal. These concerns may result in a range of shifting moods, from sudden unexplainable sadness to quick, short bursts of anger over the most trivial things.

Postpartum Blues

Your baby is born and there is a wonderul sense of accomplishment and excitement, with best wishes and congratulations from friends and relatives. Then several days after the birth, the emotional letdown hits you and the sense of inadequacy to cope, the fatigue, and irritability are back. It's the postpartum "blues," or depression, and, as before, it signals a period of adjustment, thankfully in most cases lasting only a few days.

Arriving home, the new mother has to take on the regular duties of daily life, coping with the needs of the new baby for feedings and diaper changes day and night and the desire of friends and family to come see the new addition. At the same time it takes weeks for the new mother to regain her full strength and energy. If it is possible for the baby's father to take time off from work, he can be very helpful during the first week or two after the mother and baby come home from the hospital. If he cannot be available, help from a relative or friend or someone hired can make a big difference during this period of adjustment.

Our purpose here is not to create the impression that the experience of pregnancy is one of exhaustion, irritability, and emotional turmoil. It is not. And yet these factors do play a part, and our point is that if you experience them, don't be thrown by them, but know that they are a normal part of the experience.

Recommendations

In fact, there are certain things that you, the expectant mother, can do that will help you adjust to and understand the feelings you may be experiencing during and following pregnancy. First, we urge you to turn to this book to help you understand those changes that may be worrisome to you. Being thoroughly informed is one of the best preventions for anxiety and feelings of inadequacy. Being informed also helps cope with those temporary periods of depression that are so commonly associated with pregnancy. Second, discuss freely with your doctor and your husband or partner those things that may be bothering you. Your doctor can be most helpful when truly aware of the feelings you are experiencing and the concerns you have. Do not feel that you are taking up too much time or asking silly questions. In our experience in taking care of literally thousands of pregnant women, we have come to feel that there are no foolish or unnecessary questions. Your doctor will sense your needs and be able to help you understand your feelings.

Avoid taking on tasks that are unimportant or excessively demanding and don't take on duties that need not actually be yours, such as caring for relatives or close friends. These may lead to frustrations and aggravation of any emotional stresses you may be undergoing. Try to evaluate the necessity of any work that may be overloading you and leading to excessive fatigue or tiredness. An assessment of this type may indicate that some tasks that you felt were important could actually be avoided or deferred. Correspondingly, you should be sure you get adequate rest and sleep. These are most important factors in easing stress and anxiety.

Finally, do not cut out your usual interests and activities. At the same time, be careful about taking on new responsibilities and activities. Thus, while it is quite proper for one who is a regular jogger to continue this activity in pregnancy, it is not something that should be taken up as a new form of exercise by the pregnant patient who has not been doing it regularly prior to pregnancy. This applies to many other physical activities and exercises as well.

Taking these suggested steps will not eliminate the emotional stresses associated with pregnancy, but they will certainly make it much easier for you to cope with them.

5

NUTRITION AND HEALTH
IN PREGNANCY

Since, in a certain real sense, we are what we eat, it is hard to think of anything much more important in our daily routine than the choosing and preparing of our food. It is fortunate that so many people are aware of the basic elements of nutrition, but it is well to remember also the importance of the individual advice of your physician in this matter, both for your own sake and for the baby's. While the suggestions in this chapter regarding your food planning and other health routines are applicable in most cases, there are circumstances in which the physician may well be justified in offering different advice based on thorough knowledge of your individual situation. For your own further reading you may wish to have an information booklet prepared by the American College of Obstetricians and Gynecologists entitled *Food, Pregnancy and Family Health*, which can be helpful in planning your daily meal guide in pregnancy and lactation. To obtain it, write ACOG, 409 Twelfth Street S.W., Washington, D.C. 20024–2188. You may also wish to write the Consumer Information Center, Pueblo, Colorado 81009, for information on nutritional pamphlets available from the federal government.

Quality and Quantity of Food

The old saying that a pregnant woman must eat for two is one of those half-truths that has done far more harm than good. The fallacy lies in the implication that a great increase is necessary in the *quantity* of food eaten. This is quite wrong, and if heeded will result in appalling gains of fat that may never be lost. If viewed from the standpoint of the *quality* of the diet, the old saying has much to recommend it, since the foods eaten in pregnancy must not only meet the requirements of the mother's tissues but also include a wide variety of food elements (particularly protein, minerals, and vitamins) necessary for the building of the baby's body.

The amount of food consumed by the pregnant woman should be the amount she has been accustomed to eating when not pregnant, for there is no reason to believe that any appreciable increase in the total quantity of food is necessary in pregnancy. To be sure, the growing fetus and enlarging uterus represent an additional amount of tissue to be nourished but this tends to be counterbalanced by the reduction in muscular activity that advancing pregnancy entails. As you know, the energy-producing value of food is expressed in calories; that is, in heat units that indicate the amount of energy a given food furnishes as it is burned in the body. The Food and Nutrition Board of the National Academy of Sciences–National Research Council recommends 2,300 to 2,400 calories per day in pregnancy (for women eighteen to thirty-five years old) — only 300 to 400 calories more than for the moderately active nonpregnant woman (see Appendix 3 for calorie chart). Of special importance is the fact that this board advises a substantial increase in the amount of protein eaten during pregnancy — roughly an additional 20 to 30 grams per day, or a total of 75 grams.

During the early months of pregnancy the appetite is likely to be poor, and in some instances there is an actual distaste for food. When nausea militates still further against adequate food intake there is some danger that dietary deficiencies may develop. As will be discussed in detail when we consider the whole problem of nausea (pages 111–113), every effort should be made to work out some form of dietary regimen during this period to supply the most important food elements, even though the total quantity of food eaten is temporarily minimal. After the third month the appetite usually increases and sometimes becomes voracious, which can be a genuine annoyance. While many subterfuges have been recommended to meet this situation, a certain degree of self-restraint is an essential ingredient in most of them and must be cultivated in some way, at least to the extent of keeping to a definite diet plan and avoiding any snacks and beverages not provided for in the plan. Fatty foods and sweets especially should be curtailed. At meals, of course, there is no limit to the amount of vegetables such as lettuce, tomatoes, celery, string beans, carrots, and beets, and fruits rich in vitamin C that may be eaten, and by increasing the quantity of such foods to several times the amount ordinarily taken, it is usually possible to maintain a comfortable fullness without gaining abnormally in weight.

On the other hand, attempts to reduce food intake to exceedingly low levels are unwarranted and may even be harmful. In general, such reducing diets have no place in the health program of the normal pregnant woman, but if she is markedly overweight or gaining very rapidly, some type of low-calorie diet may be prescribed by the physician. For the benefit of such patients the whole problem of weight considerations in pregnancy is discussed in detail later (see chapter 6).

If you have been accustomed to a varied diet, rich in natural foods such as milk, eggs, fruits, green vegetables, and meat, little if any alteration is needed during pregnancy. You should review, nevertheless, the following food groups to make certain that each is represented in your diet each day.

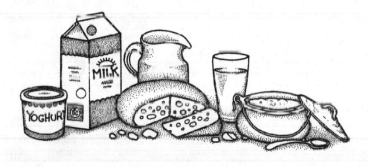

MILK AND MILK PRODUCTS
(Four or more cups daily, including miscellaneous uses or equivalents)

Milk is invaluable to the pregnant woman for a number of reasons. In the first place, it contains all the different kinds of mineral elements the fetal skeleton needs. For instance, its high content of calcium and phosphorus makes it a very valuable food for good growth of bone and teeth; it provides these minerals, moreover, in just the correct proportions and in a digestible form that permits their complete utilization by both mother and child. Second, it is an excellent source of protein, our tissue-building material. The particular proteins present in milk not only are unexcelled in their ability to promote tissue growth but are also the most readily digested and easily absorbed of all food proteins. Finally, milk contains some of all of the vitamins, particularly vitamin A (often with added A or D), and safeguards the development of the fetus.

In view of these facts, a total of one quart (four cups) of milk daily should be at the top of your dietary list. At least two eight-ounce glasses a day (one pint) should be taken as such, and the rest, if you prefer, may be in soups, custards and other puddings, on cereal, in cooked dishes, and so on. Evaporated milk and dried milk are widely used because of their convenience and economy. Nonfat (skim) milk may be used in place of whole fresh milk, to avoid unnecessary fat.

If you don't like milk, try mixing it with a flavor you like — a few drops of vanilla, a half-teaspoon of honey, or a scattering of nutmeg and cinnamon. Since half of the daily amount can be disguised in various dishes (as noted above), and dry milk is easily added to a wide range of recipes, that may meet your difficulty. The various forms of calcium available in tablets might seem to be a satisfactory substitute for the calcium of milk. Although this is doubtless true of some of these products, the calcium in this form has been known, in some instances, to pass through the intestines unchanged; in other words, calcium taken in tablet form might not be absorbed and therefore cannot be regarded as an absolutely dependable substitute for that in milk.

From a theoretical standpoint, the only acceptable substitutes for milk are yogurt, which adds helpful bacteria to the food values of whole milk, and cheese, which contains in concentrated form all the important food elements of milk, with the exception of milk sugar. Because it is such a concentrated food, however, cheese must be eaten with restraint. One ounce of Cheddar, American, or Swiss cheese (a cube about an inch and a quarter thick) contains approximately the same amount of calcium, phosphorus, proteins, and vitamins as an eight-ounce glass of whole milk. Such cheeses may be used sparingly, let us say an ounce or two a day, to replace a portion of the milk recommended, or more may be used if you are not eating meat. Cottage cheese, though rich in protein, is in respect to calcium not a satisfactory substitute for milk, since for the amount of calcium present in half a glass of milk you would need about five tablespoons of cottage cheese. Whole-milk cheese is a good source of vitamin A.

If you wish to avoid milk because of a weight control factor, use skim milk. It must be remembered that excessive weight gain can result from eating more food than is needed; that is, consuming more calories than the energy requirements call for. If gain is excessive, then, it is not the milk that is at fault, but added foods such as extra snacks or rich desserts. Protein, not sweets or unnecessary starches, should be the basic food in pregnancy, for no other can serve so well as the foundation of a complete diet.

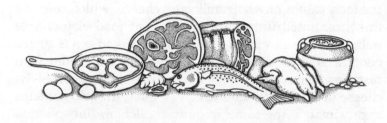

EGGS, MEAT, FISH, POULTRY, DRIED BEANS AND PEAS, AND NUTS
(Two or more servings daily)

As stated on pages 59–60, the Food and Nutrition Board of the National Research Council recommends a substantial increase in the amount of protein in the diet during pregnancy. The total quantity advised is 75 grams a day, the greater part of which is supplied by one or two eggs, a quart of milk (or a pint of milk and the equivalent of another pint), a serving of meat, fish, or poultry (or a dish made with dried beans, peas, or lentils as an extender or alternative to the meat, fish, or poultry), with the remainder furnished by vegetables and fruits, brown cereals, and whole-grain or enriched bread.

One egg should be included in the menu each day, unless you have a high cholesterol value, since the yolks in particular are a rich source of iron and vitamins.

Since we are again stressing the desirability of an iron-rich food in the diet of the pregnant woman, it may be well to explain the reason. The function of iron in the body is exceedingly important, for it is an essential element in the oxygen-carrying material of the red blood cells, hemoglobin. This is the substance that makes blood red and gives to cheeks their ruddiness; when we say that a person is pale or anemic-looking, we mean that the blood is low in this iron-containing pigment, hemoglobin. Despite the importance of iron, the amount present in the body is small, about a tenth of an ounce in a full-grown healthy person. The iron needs must be met day by day in the diet. Now, throughout the latter part of pregnancy the fetus, unlike the adult, stores iron in its liver for future use; this is wise planning on nature's part, since the baby will have to subsist after birth largely on milk, which is low in iron. Since the fetus also requires iron for building red blood cells, the demand imposed on the mother for this mineral is so great that about a third of pregnant women develop some degree of anemia through lack of it. The necessity for ample amounts of iron-containing foods in pregnancy, therefore, cannot be overemphasized. While the iron supplied by one egg represents only one tenth of the total daily need, this form of iron is assimilated by the body with particular ease.

It is our custom to recommend one serving of lean meat daily and to suggest that liver, varied by heart or kidney if you like, be eaten at least once a week. These meats differ considerably in nutritive value from the muscle tissue so generally preferred by Americans. They are not only exceedingly rich in iron and copper, which is necessary for the utilization of iron, but furnish certain essential substances needed for the building of red blood cells; at the same time they are abundantly supplied with important vitamins. The amount of liver eaten at one time need not be large; for instance, one small piece three inches square and a half-inch thick contains more iron than two eggs. Oysters are excelled only by liver as a source of blood-building materials and may be substituted for liver. Liver and egg yolk are also high sources of cholesterol, which some women may need to avoid.

Because of the tendency to develop anemia in pregnancy and the difficulty of meeting iron needs by natural foods, many physicians make it a routine to prescribe an iron compound in the form of capsules or tablets for daily ingestion. Various vitamins are often included in the capsule.

Dried beans and peas, lentils, whole-grain or enriched grain products, and nuts are also good sources of iron as well as of other minerals and vitamins. In addition they are the best plant sources of protein, and are well worth using in your meal plans even if you feel you do not need their advantage of economy, since a mixture of plant-derived and animal-derived proteins at each meal is your best guarantee of obtaining all the essential amino acids from your daily protein supply. (Amino acids are the building blocks for protein in our bodies. The eight "essential" amino acids must be supplied by our diet, since the body cannot otherwise supply them.)

Dried beans, peas, and lentils, as well as many forms of whole grains, make excellent main dishes, which are sometimes enhanced by the addition of such animal-derived protein sources as eggs, cheese, milk, or bits of leftover meat, fish, or poultry. Dried soybeans rank very high in quantity and quality of protein and other nutrients, and can be used in many different forms and ways. Nuts added to salads or used as a garnish with other dishes will supply good nutritive value, but are so high in calories that caution is advised. The same is true of peanut butter, an excellent and nutritious protein-supplying meal stretcher, especially in combination with milk or cheese, but one that also supplies 95 calories per tablespoon.

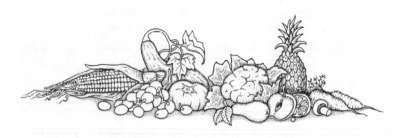

VEGETABLES AND FRUITS
(For recommended daily servings, see below)

The vitamins and minerals our bodies need are widely distributed in vegetables and fruits, which are major sources for many of them, and these are also the foods we most count on for variety and attractiveness in our meals. To benefit from different nutrients in different fruits and vegetables, use as wide a range of them in your meal plans as is practical. Canned and frozen varieties may be used in place of fresh when you like; the vitamin content is often higher than that of vegetables cooked at home. On the other hand, some food values are reduced in such processing, so eat fresh fruits and vegetables as much as you can.

Vegetable cooking should be brief, with a minimum of water. The vegetable should be tender when done but still crisp and flavorful. Steam-cooking is a good method for most vegetables. Bring a quarter-inch to half-inch of water to a boil in a heavy saucepan with a tight-fitting lid, drop in the prepared vegetable, cover, and allow to steam gently over medium heat until tender. Put greens in the pot with only the water clinging to them from washing, and cut larger vegetables for quicker cooking. Check frequently; the method is quick, but scorching is possible if the water wholly evaporates. If any water is left, drink it or use it in soups, sauces, casseroles, breads, and so on — it is rich in nutrients.

Many vegetables besides the usual salad ingredients may be eaten raw as well as cooked (broccoli, spinach, carrots, zucchini, and others), which can add still more variety to your diet. Whether you are serving a fresh vegetable raw or cooked, for the sake of its appearance as well as its nutrient content, try to (1) eat it soon after gathering or buying it; (2) keep it in the refrigerator crisping section until use; (3) delay cutting, slicing, shredding, or peeling until the last minute; and (4) if cooking, do so as near serving time as you can.

In addition to their value as nutrient agents, fruits and vegetables deserve an important place in our diet because they, along with the whole-grain group, increase the bulk of the bowel content, which stimulates the eliminative action of the intestine.

Recommended Daily Servings

As to how much is a good daily allowance of fruits and vegetables, you can feel free to eat as much as you like unless your own experience, or your doctor's advice, indicates otherwise. You will need to consider also the matter of calories, since some fruits and vegetables are fairly high in them and might be better assigned to an otherwise low-calorie meal than to an already high-calorie one. A good rule is to eat every day at least one good serving from the first list (*Especially for Vitamin A*); at least two from the

second list (*Especially for Vitamin C*); and at least two other
servings from the third list or from all three lists or from
among fruits and vegetables not listed at all (since we cannot cover all the variety of these categories that might be
available to you). In addition, or as part of the servings,
you will no doubt be using small quantities of vegetables
or fruits as garnishes for other dishes, in salads, as raw
vegetable snacks, and so on.

Especially for Vitamin A
(Dark green and deep yellow vegetables; those starred
are particularly high in iron and vitamin content). *One or
more servings daily.*

Asparagus (green)
Beans (green lima)
Beans (green snap)
*Beet greens
*Broccoli
Brussels sprouts
Cabbage (greens)
Carrots
*Chard
*Collards
*Dandelion greens
Endive (curly; also called
    chicory)
Escarole

*Kale
Lettuce (leaf)
*Mustard greens
Okra
Peas (green)
Peppers (green and red)
Pumpkin
*Spinach
Squash (winter yellow:
    butternut, acorn,
    Hubbard)
Sweet potatoes
*Turnip greens

As rich sources of vitamin A, iron, and other vitamins
and minerals, the dark green and deep yellow vegetables are especially important in menus for the pregnant
woman, and especially the crisp green vegetables. You'll

find good vitamin A content in some fruits too — apricots, the orange-fleshed cantaloupes, yellow-fleshed peaches, and papayas.

Especially for Vitamin C
(Citrus fruits and other sources). *Two or more servings daily.*

Citrus fruits: grapefruit, kumquats, lemons, limes, oranges, tangerines, and their juices
Other fresh (raw) fruits: cantaloupe (muskmelon), papaya, pineapple, strawberries
Tomatoes and tomato juice
Other vegetables: broccoli, brussels sprouts, raw cabbage, greens, raw green peppers, potatoes, raw turnip
NOTE: A large serving of the vegetables in this group can be substituted for the fruits

Not until late in the eighteenth century did the importance of fresh fruits and vegetables in the diet begin to be appreciated, and as a consequence of the lack of knowledge, tens of thousands of people died, especially men at sea. Back in the days when intrepid navigators were exploring uncharted seas in year-long voyages, perishable goods such as fruit, milk, eggs, and green vegetables had no place on such extended cruises, and the fare was restricted to dried and salty foods. Although hidden reefs and icebergs were constant dangers, more deadly than these was an insidious disease that afflicted the men after a few months at sea, a malady characterized by growing listlessness, bone pains, and swollen, bleeding gums. The disease became known as scurvy. The ravages of scurvy were such that three-quarters of a ship's crew often succumbed; but not until the eighteenth century was it finally discovered that fresh fruits and vegetables would cure and prevent the disease. In 1795 the British navy began rationing out lemon juice daily on long voyages. Later the ration was changed to lime juice, and it was because of this dole that English sailors began to be called "limeys." Here, also, is the genesis of the name Limehouse — the waterfront district in London where the fruit was stored.

We know now that these sailors died because a certain substance necessary for life was absent from their diet; this substance, vitamin C or ascorbic acid, is found particularly in fresh fruits. We might mention other dire and fatal diseases that result when certain other vitamins are withheld completely, but today we seldom see examples of complete vitamin deprivation in the United States. We do see, however, some cases of partial vitamin deficiency, and these are particularly insidious because less readily recognized. There is no evidence (for the person eating a normal diet) that supplements of vitamins and minerals are necessary during pregnancy, except for iron and possibly folate or vitamin B_6.

Fruits, particularly oranges, lemons, and grapefruit, are not only rich sources of vitamin C but also contain liberal amounts of other important vitamins. From a nutritional standpoint tomatoes fall into this same group and may be substituted for fruits as desired. Another excellent and usually less expensive source of vitamin C is raw cabbage, which as coleslaw may be the foundation for many an appetizing combination. Peaches, plums, pineapples, and apricots are but a few of the fruits that may be combined with leaf lettuce, watercress, and other greens, or with shredded raw cabbage, to yield vitamin-rich, health-giving dishes with unsurpassed flavors. The noted beauty authority Madame Helena Rubinstein stressed again and again in her writings that beauty is not "skin deep" but depends on vibrant internal health. Clear skin, glistening hair, and all that goes with the glamour and vitality of youth, she points out, are to be found *par excellence* in a diet rich in raw fruits and vegetables. During pregnancy, when the need for vitamins and minerals is greatly increased, these raw foods become doubly necessary.

Other Vegetables and Fruits: Two or more servings daily.

Artichokes	Apples
Beans (yellow snap)	Avocados
Beets	Bananas
Cabbage (red; white)	Berries
Cauliflower	Cherries
Celery	Cranberries
Corn (sweet)	Currants
Cucumbers	Dates
Eggplant	Figs
Leeks	Grapes
Lettuce (head)	Pears
Mushrooms	Persimmons
Onions	Pineapple and pineapple
Parsnips	juice (canned)
Radishes	Plums
Rutabagas	Prunes
Salsify (oyster plant)	Raisins
Sauerkraut	Rhubarb
Squash (summer: yellow	Watermelon
or green, including	
zucchini)	

All of these vegetables and fruits contribute worthwhile amounts of minerals and vitamins, introduce variety into the diet, and because of their bulk help satisfy the appetite.

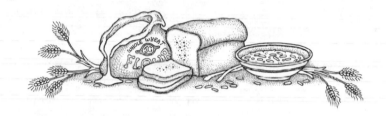

WHOLE-WHEAT OR OTHER WHOLE-GRAIN OR ENRICHED BREADS AND CEREALS *(Every day)*

Breads and flours: all the bread types (quick or yeast-raised loaf breads, muffins, rolls, biscuits, pancakes, crackers, low-calorie breads) made with whole-wheat flour, other whole-grain flours, enriched flour, or any mixture of these, including also oatmeal or rolled oats, whole-grain cornmeal, wheat germ, and (though not strictly in this category) soy flour

Breakfast cereals: whole-grain or enriched, dry or to be cooked, made with barley, buckwheat, corn, oats, rice, rye, wheat, and other cereal, either whole-grain or re-stored

Lunch or dinner dishes: pilafs, spoon breads, macaroni and cheese, and many others made with whole-grain or enriched cereal products such as grits, rice (brown or converted), bulgur or wheat pilaf, cornmeal, egg noodles, and other enriched pastas

Prior to 1830 wheat flour was obtained simply by grinding the whole grain between stones. As a result the bread in those days contained both the germ and the outer shell (bran) of the wheat kernel. It was brown in color, naturally, and somewhat coarser in texture than most of the bread we eat today, but it was so nutritious and health-building that our ancestors, you remember, called it the "staff of life." The invention of the roller mill for the manufacture of wheat flour, about 1830, appeared to mark a great advance. By eliminating the germ and the shell, it made possible the production of flour that was less subject to deterioration than whole-wheat and consequently more suitable for commerce; the flour, moreover, was white in color and fine in consistency, qualities that not only appealed to the eye but suggested greater purity. The new process was a sweeping commercial success, and white bread became the most important staple of the American diet.

Then — not so long ago — physicians suffered a rude awakening in learning that these refinements in milling had deprived bread of some of its most important nutritive constituents. Both the germ and the shell of the wheat kernel are rich in iron, protein, and essential vitamins such as the B vitamins and vitamin E. Deficiency in certain of the B vitamins reveals itself principally by digestive disturbances and by inflammation and degeneration of the nerves, but these degenerative diseases are rarely seen in the United States today. From the viewpoint of the expectant mother, however, it is even more important to know that during pregnancy more of the B vitamins are required to saturate the body than are needed in the nonpregnant state. This need for additional B vitamins can almost always be accommodated by attention to the diet as described here, although often supplements are given.

It has been estimated that modern milling methods do away with more than 90 percent of the B vitamins present in the old stone-ground flour. An almost ludicrous example of the inadequacy of modern diets in this respect was a British study of the 1930s comparing the nutritive value of the then current London diet with that of the rations specified in the 1830s by the Poor Law of London. The food penuriously doled out to the indigent in 1838 turned out to contain twice the quantity of B vitamins present in the diet of the highest income groups of London in 1937.

Despite the widespread enrichment of flours and cereal products with iron and B vitamins, and the increased availability of whole-grain products, the conclusion seems inescapable that a large fraction of our population subsists on diets of borderline adequacy in respect to the B vitamins. If American diets as a whole are frequently unsatisfactory in this regard, as physicians and nutritionists now believe, they are particularly inadequate to meet the increased needs during pregnancy. Accordingly, whole-wheat bread and flour, and other whole-grain breads and flours, should replace most of the white bread and flour in your diet, insofar as is possible. Check labels to make sure the white flour, white bread, and any other flour items you may buy are enriched, and check labels on all cereal products so you will know the calorie count and the nutritive value of the product.

To further increase your intake of these essential B vitamins — and of the minerals and vitamin E in whole-grain cereals — seize the opportunity at breakfast to eat still more whole-grain products such as rolled oats, shredded wheat, and other brown cereals; also explore opportunities for serving whole-grain dishes at other meals. (For vitamin E, see also page 77, under Fats.)

Summary: Daily Minimum from the Food Groups

One or more items from each of the following food groups, in the following minimum quantities.

1. *Milk and milk products (except butter).* One quart, or one pint (or more) with the rest of the quart in the form of equivalents, such as cheese or yogurt.

2. *Eggs, meat, fish, poultry, dried beans and peas, and nuts.* One egg, better two. One serving of lean meat or poultry or fish, varied by dishes made with dried beans or peas, and including liver once or more weekly if possible. Occasional use of nuts, if you like.

3. *Vegetables and fruits.* One serving from the first list (dark green and deep yellow vegetables and fruits, especially for vitamin A). Two servings from the second list (citrus fruits, tomatoes, and other fruits and vegetables, especially for vitamin C). Two servings from the third list or a combination of lists.

4. *Whole-wheat or other whole-grain or enriched breads and*

cereals. Use in different forms every day (at least two servings), with emphasis on whole-wheat or other whole-grain products.

The above are basic protective foods designed to safeguard you and your baby, and should be regarded as obligatory. They furnish ordinarily, however, only about two-thirds of your daily pregnancy requirements. The makeup of the remaining third rests entirely with you, provided the total amount does not exceed your usual consumption. The best advice is to stay as much as possible within the four groups and to plan meals with plenty of variety, suiting your own and your family's tastes and keeping an eye on your weight. A few more food notes:

Fats and Oils

Fat is essential in the diet, but since it pervades other foods no special effort is usually needed to supply it. Use just enough butter, margarine, or vegetable oils for pleasant seasoning; no more — these, and cooking fats, are very high in calories. Butter and margarine are rich in vitamin A, but there are other sources of this vitamin (see pages 69–70). Vegetable oils and margarine are important sources of vitamin E, along with salad dressings, whole-grain cereals, and peanuts. As much as possible, use polyunsaturated fats.

Sugars

Sugars and the various sugar syrups are generally high in calories and low in nourishment, though corn and sorghum syrups and brown sugar do contain calcium and iron. Depend as much as you can on the natural sweetness of whole grains, fruits, and vegetables, and remember that most dry cereals are already supplied with extra sugar.

Desserts

The best dessert for nutritional balance and delicious taste is probably the long-time favorite of fresh fruit, accompanied if you wish by a little cheese and a few nuts. But many others can fit well into your menus, as long as you are alert to the need for nutritional value in dessert too, and generally avoid candies, layer cakes, fudge sauce, and the like except for occasional samples if your weight is no problem.

Low-Calorie Substitutes

These can be useful but need careful assessment in a nutrition plan. Check with your doctor before deciding to use (or continue) such substitutes, and above all avoid any form of crash dieting if you are concerned about your weight (see chapter 6).

Iodine

Although only infinitesimal quantities of iodine are needed by the body, a small amount is necessary for the health of mother and baby alike. This may be ensured by eating seafood twice a week or by the use of iodized salt. In some localities in the United States, the water and soil have lost their iodine, and consequently the foods grown in these regions may provide inadequate amounts. Not infrequently doctors in these localities prescribe small amounts of iodine for expectant mothers, but iodine should only be taken upon the advice and under the immediate supervision of a physician. Excess iodine can cause goiter, or enlargement of the thyroid gland, in the fetus. Do not use cough medicines containing iodine.

Foods to Avoid

It is only common sense to avoid any article of diet that you know disagrees with you. During pregnancy the stomach and other digestive organs are encroached upon by the growing uterus and will often not tolerate foods that in nonpregnancy cause no difficulty. The following articles of diet are common offenders: rich foods and condiments of all sorts, fried foods, sausage, smoked or salt fish, and rich pastries. You may even find that some of the foods recommended in the first list under Group 3 (dark green and deep yellow vegetables and fruits) may at first prove upsetting. If so, it is very probable that the digestive tract has become so pampered by artificially prepared foods that at the outset it is unable to stand foods in their natural state. Under such circumstances there is no time so good as the present to swing over to correct eating habits. This must be done gradually, however, increasing little by little the amount of raw foods taken, remembering always that their digestibility is immeasurably increased by prolonged chewing.

The excessive use of salt during pregnancy should be avoided. In the first place, the amount of salt consumed by the average person is usually in excess of requirements. Second, even if *no* salt were added to foods either in the kitchen or at the table, this mineral is so widely distributed in food materials that the likelihood of shortage would be exceedingly remote. Finally, there is a definite relationship between the amount of salt eaten and the amount of water retained by the body; that is, the greater the salt intake the greater the tendency of tissues to absorb water. The tissues of the pregnant woman show a particular eagerness for water, as can be seen by the tendency of the face and fingers to become puffy, and if, added to this tendency, there is an excess of salt in the diet, the tissues may become swollen. In normal pregnancy, salt, like fluids, should be neither excessively restricted nor markedly increased. If you are using — or plan to use — a salt substitute, check with your physician.

Fluids

Six glasses of water should be taken daily, and more in hot weather. An ample fluid intake in pregnancy seems to flush out the kidneys and prevent infections of these organs that are not uncommon at this time.

Gain in Weight

During the first three and a half months of pregnancy the maternal weight is usually stationary and may show a slight loss secondary to nausea. During the latter two-thirds of pregnancy, however, there is a steady gain, over some twenty-four weeks, which averages about a pound a week. The greater part of this twenty-four-pound increase is quite understandable, as shown by the following figures:

Baby	7 pounds
Afterbirth	1
Amniotic fluid	1½
Increase in weight of uterus	2
Increase in blood	3
Increase in weight of breasts	1½
	16 pounds

The remaining eight pounds represent in part general accumulation of fat and in part the increased amount of fluid that tissues tend to retain at this time. Gains between twenty-two and twenty-seven pounds are natural and in keeping with good health; they are usually lost, moreover, after the baby is born. On the contrary, increases in weight of thirty pounds and more are undesirable for a number of reasons. In the first place, they include unnecessary poundage for the muscles of the legs and back to carry about, and this suddenly imposed strain is a common cause of backache and pain in the legs. You will usually feel much better if you keep your weight gain about twenty-five pounds over your ideal or standard weight. Second, some complications of pregnancy and labor are associated with excessive weight gain. In other words, you and your baby will be healthier and safer if you follow this advice. Finally, huge accumulations of fat are likely to be permanent acquisitions that can be removed only by the most rigorous dieting and exercise. You will feel much better if you adhere to the rule of keeping weight between twenty-five and thirty pounds above your proper weight.

The grid shown in Figure 7 supplies a handy method of checking your own weight advances, which will be helpful in guiding your diet and progress. Although some variations from the graph occur in perfectly normal pregnancies, marked deviations should be discussed with your doctor. The chart is intended only as a helpful guide in seeking good nutritional patterns during your pregnancy. As discussed previously, your pre-pregnancy weight will have obvious considerations in determining your optimal weight advances. Your physician will advise you regarding nutritional requirements in your particular case. (For more on weight in pregnancy see chapter 6.)

General Health Considerations in Pregnancy

Using the Prenatal Weight Gain Chart (opposite page)
The chart can be used to mark your own weight gain in pregnancy; the line already on the chart is the *average* weight gain in pregnancy. Each square represents one week (numbers from left to right) and one pound (numbers from the baseline to the top). The squares below the baseline are for recording weight loss.

Check with your doctor about any aspect of the chart you need help with. For your convenience, we include the following table of standard weights (as drawn from the Metropolitan Life Insurance Company Actuarial Tables) so that you can compare your own weight at the start of pregnancy with the figure given here. Weigh yourself with shoes as normally worn. The figures are for medium body build, and anyone under the age of twenty-five should deduct one pound for each year under. For example, if your height without shoes is five feet and four inches, and you are twenty-one years old: 5'4" + 1 = 5'5" (128 pounds); and 128 pounds − 4 = 124 pounds (your standard weight).

Standard Weights
(in pounds)
(height without shoes plus 1 inch)

4'10" = 104	5'3" = 118	5'8" = 140
4'11" = 107	5'4" = 123	5'9" = 144
5'0" = 110	5'5" = 128	5'10" = 148
5'1" = 113	5'6" = 132	5'11" = 152
5'2" = 116	5'7" = 136	6'0" = 156

PRENATAL WEIGHT GAIN GRID

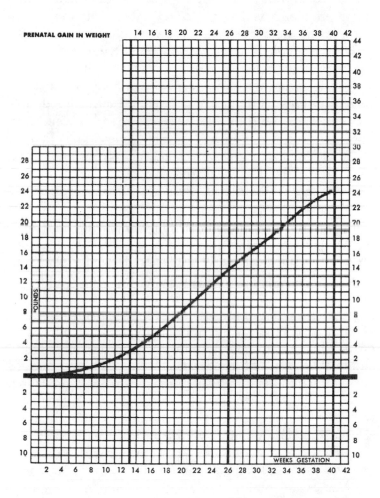

FIGURE 7. Prenatal weight gain grid. Reprinted with permission from *Clinical Obstetrics* 1953, J. B. Lippincott and Co.

Clothing

It is probably obvious that the first requirement for clothing in pregnancy is that it be comfortable. With the obliteration of the waistline by the growing uterus at about the fifth month, it is increasingly difficult to hang clothes from the hips, and much of what you wear will have to be suspended from the shoulders. Constriction of the abdomen interferes with your breathing and may impede free movement of the baby. For these reasons, as well as for your own comfort, you will probably like clothes that are full and flowing. However, maternity skirts and slacks have an expandable waistband that can be adjusted to a level just above the uterus, thus sparing any pressure on that organ.

As at any other time, it is important for a pregnant woman to dress well, for her own sense of self-esteem. But dressing attractively and being generally well-groomed in pregnancy can also be an expression of pride in your condition, a celebration of your changing body. There is now a wide variety of styles of maternity clothing to choose from, whether you buy any specialized pregnancy clothes you need or make them. In addition, you have a strong natural ally in the matter of appearance since, for some reason, during the middle months of pregnancy women develop a special radiance, suggesting an inner glow, which makes whatever you have chosen to wear look most becoming.

From the standpoint of your physical well-being there are only a few precautions to be kept in mind. Whatever you wear should keep you comfortably warm, but American homes are typically at such regulated temperatures that probably no special effort will be necessary. However, when you are out of doors on cold or wet days, every care should be taken to prevent soaking or chilling.

Leg constriction. Since the growing uterus not only bulges forward but also presses backward against the veins that drain blood from the legs, the circulation in the lower extremities is often sluggish in pregnancy. This is the reason for swelling of the ankles so often seen during the later weeks. It is important that panty hose be well fitting and nonconstrictive, so as not to obstruct still further the return flow of blood from the legs. Support stockings are recommended if you are on your feet a good deal. Knee-high hose should be avoided.

Shoes. From the standpoint of weight distribution, the pregnant woman is not unlike a person carrying a twelve-pound basket pressed against the abdomen. In order to support the weight and maintain equilibrium, it is necessary to tilt the torso backward. The resultant swayback posture puts additional strain on the muscles of the abdomen, back, and thighs, and accounts for many of the muscular aches that sometimes accompany the later weeks of pregnancy. Since high heels accentuate the swayback posture, they may cause, or aggravate, muscular cramps in these regions as pregnancy progresses. The second objection to high heels is their tendency to cause accidents, either trip-ups or ankle-turnings, both of which usually mean a fall. In view of these facts, excessively high heels, and very high soles as well, are to be avoided. The generally most satisfactory shoe has a low heel which is broad enough to support your increased weight, and has a full back rather than a sling. Since there is a slight tendency for the feet to swell in the evenings as pregnancy advances, it is well to purchase shoes a trifle larger than usual. In flat footwear, the worst dangers are from slippery soles or flopping sandals, which should be avoided.

Maternity girdle. The primary purpose of a maternity girdle is to promote your comfort during the latter months of pregnancy. For most women it is usually unnecessary and may prove a hindrance to comfort rather than a help, particularly in warm weather. A number of expectant mothers, however, find such a garment a distinct aid after the fifth month, particularly women who have had previous children. Its function is to support the growing uterus from below without compressing it and without exerting pressure on the upper abdomen, thus allowing ample room for deep breathing and for the baby's activity. It also provides a stay for the back and in this way relieves the back muscles of a certain amount of strain. Needless to say, any girdle should be fitted by a competent person and should be of a type in keeping with your size and build.

During the first half of pregnancy an ordinary elastic girdle without stays may contribute to your comfort, especially if you have been accustomed to wearing one. But it is not necessary and most expectant mothers do not need this support.

Brassiere. The breasts are much more comfortable when supported by a brassiere of the uplift or sling type that lifts each breast upward and inward. Anything that flattens the breast is injurious and should never be worn.

Bathing

Although it is important at any time for the bathtub or shower stall to have a good nonslip surface, it is especially important as pregnancy advances, since equilibrium is likely to be uncertain at this time and there is a danger of losing one's footing in the slippery tub and falling. Extra care should be taken getting in and out of the tub. Prolonged soaks in an extremely hot bath or "hot tub" should be avoided.

Teeth

The old saying "For every child a tooth" is based upon the belief that the fetus takes calcium from the mother's teeth. Although modern investigation refutes this contention, there is no doubt that some women do suffer markedly from dental decay during pregnancy. Accordingly, the dentist should be consulted early and the recommendations followed. The old notion that dental work causes miscarriage is without basis; on the contrary, a thorough overhauling of the teeth early in pregnancy is a good preventive measure against the decay mentioned above. Extractions are preferably done under local anesthesia. Routine X rays can be postponed. Should dental X rays be necessary, your body should be shielded with a lead apron, which your dentist will provide. Meanwhile, assiduous care should be used in brushing the teeth and rinsing thoroughly after meals, and in the daily use of dental floss.

Nipples

As we have already noted, there is a tendency for the colostrum, the sticky fluid the breasts secrete in pregnancy, to cake on the nipples and cause irritation. To remove this, the nipples should be gently cleansed in the bath with a soft cloth and warm water, no soap. This may be done as often as is necessary, particular care being used to dry the nipples thoroughly afterward.

The nipples need no preparation for their functioning. Some have advised tugging gently with the thumb and fingers a dozen times at night and morning or rubbing with towels or lanolin cream, but there is no evidence that this is necessary during pregnancy.

Douches

Douches should not be taken in pregnancy unless your doctor has approved them and given specific instructions regarding them.

Sexual Intercourse

The usual sexual relations are perfectly permissible and harmless during the first eight months of pregnancy. The couple may find that varying the positions for intercourse may be more comfortable, and other forms of sexual expression may be helpful to both partners.

Some women experience contractions with intercourse during pregnancy, but the danger of infection or harm to the baby is remote. If you have a history of premature births you should consult your doctor about intercourse. In general, intercourse with deep penetration should be avoided during the last month of pregnancy.

Bowels

The bowels should preferably move once daily. At least one's normal bowel habits should be maintained. If they are not, immediate and intelligent measures should be instituted to correct the difficulty, which is an extremely common one in pregnancy. The treatment of constipation is considered in detail on pages 114–116. Diarrhea may occasionally result from iron compounds or other causes. Recurrent bouts of diarrhea should be discussed with your doctor.

Exercise

Regular exercise in the open air, even though it be no more than a half-hour's walk, should form part of your

Nutrition and Health in Pregnancy

daily routine. For everyone, probably, walking is the best type of exercise; for the pregnant woman there can be no question of its superiority. It stimulates the eliminative activity of the lungs, skin, and bowels, keeps the muscles in good condition, and promotes sleep — to say nothing of the fact that it takes you away from the house or job and fosters other interests. The amount of exercise the expectant mother can comfortably and safely carry out, however, is so related to what she has been accustomed to that it is difficult, as well as undesirable, to lay down any hard-and-fast rules. For the average woman a mile or so a day is about right, but it is advisable to divide this into several short walks rather than to push oneself to cover a definite distance. Inactivity is better than any form of activity pushed grimly to the point of fatigue. Gardening, if you are so fortunate as to have a garden, is an ideal form of exercise. Housework, although in no way a substitute for out-of-door exercise, can supply helpful forms of physical activity and may be continued with profit throughout pregnancy; it should be stopped short of fatigue, however, and in no event should include the lifting of heavy objects or any other heavy work.

Violent activity is to be avoided, particularly anything that involves jolting, sudden motion, or excessive running. Although physicians vary widely in the forms of exercises they consider acceptable in pregnancy, they usually disapprove of horseback riding, strenuous tennis, skating, and skiing — not so much by reason of the sports themselves as because of the attendant danger of falling. A good general rule to follow is that you can continue to carry on those activities to which you were accustomed before pregnancy. However, many experienced physicians hold different views on various activities and it would be a good idea to ask your own doctor's opinion about your activities and certainly on any new ones you may want to undertake.

Traveling

Anyone who has ridden several hundred miles a day in an automobile knows that the experience is fatiguing, no matter how good the roads are. Since pregnant women tend to tire easily, common sense dictates that prolonged automobile trips should be planned conservatively and your doctor's approval obtained. Travel, almost regardless of distance and type of conveyance, has no harmful effect on pregnancy. Nevertheless, because of its tiring effects, automobile travel should be interspersed with rest periods. Prolonged sitting may increase the risk of venous thrombosis (clots in the veins) of the legs, and so walking at least every two hours is recommended.

When traveling by car, good safety precautions call for the use of a seat belt. Preferably this should be of the shoulder-harness type, especially in later pregnancy. If only the lap belt is available, be certain that it is placed as low as possible, over the pelvic bones in front and on the sides when feasible.

For distances greater than several hundred miles, trains and air-conditioned buses are usually safe and comfortable vehicles. Cruises are without objection, provided there is no tendency to nausea and proper care is taken to avoid injury in rough weather.

Air travel is likewise permissible. During the last month of pregnancy some airlines request a certificate from the physician attesting that the expectant mother is in good physical condition and able to travel.

Travel to remote areas late in pregnancy is unwise for

the simple reason that many babies, as we have seen, are born earlier than the calculated date of delivery. It is a good rule throughout the last month of pregnancy to be within easy reach of the place set for your delivery. If distant travel is necessary during pregnancy, carry a copy of your prenatal record in case of emergency or unexpected early delivery.

Moving

For obvious reasons many expectant parents seize upon pregnancy as an appropriate time to move into larger quarters. Nothing entails so much hard, backbreaking labor as moving. Even though a score of movers are employed, there is a great deal to do, and even after the movers leave, you are only theoretically "moved," for there is still much arranging to do in the new home; one task leads to another endlessly, and often debilitating fatigue results. If a change of quarters is necessary, plan and pace your activities to avoid excess strain and fatigue. Allow yourself plenty of time for preparation for the move and for settling into and arranging your new home. Confine your activities to organizing and directing the efforts of friends, relatives, or professional movers in packing and unpacking. Your welfare and that of your baby demand that you be sensible about your activities on such an occasion.

Employment

The expectant mother who is employed may continue if there are no complications. If the job involves significant physical labor, it may need to be modified in the last few months. Following delivery, six weeks are needed for the reproductive organs to return to normal, for the mother to regain her full strength, and for the baby to get a good start. Usually your doctor will prefer that you make no commitments about returning to work until the baby is from six to eight weeks old.

Rest

During the early months of pregnancy many women experience an almost uncontrollable desire to sleep, a good hint that more rest is required at this time. In addition to the usual amount of sleep at night, let us say eight to nine hours, it is desirable if possible for the expectant mother to lie down for an hour every afternoon, ideally on the left side, with shoes off and clothing loosened. If you sleep, fine; if not, you will feel more refreshed after an hour of complete relaxation. During the last few weeks a similar rest may also be taken in the morning. Rest is not only a psychological support; it is beneficial in the elimination of excess fluids by the kidneys and in other psychological ways.

Smoking

It is known that smoking is harmful to one's health regardless of pregnancy. If at all possible, smoking should be avoided by pregnant women. Extensive studies have shown that the newborn infants of mothers who smoke tend to weigh less than those of mothers who do not smoke. Also, nicotine has a constricting effect on the small blood vessels and may interfere with the circulation to the uterus and placenta. It is therefore important that smoking be eliminated, or at least curtailed to the greatest degree possible. If you are a smoker, consult with your physician about the best way for you to deal with your smoking.

Caffeine

There is no known harm from up to three cups of coffee per day in pregnancy. Caffeine is present in many sources, however, including colas, chocolate, and cocoa, as well as in coffee and tea, and excessive consumption should be avoided.

Alcohol

Infants of mothers who drink heavily during pregnancy have developed the "fetal alcohol syndrome" consisting of mental retardation, poor growth, and facial abnormalities. Although it is unlikely that an occasional drink is harmful, the safe level of alcohol consumption during pregnancy has not been determined. Therefore, it is advisable to limit alcohol intake during pregnancy to only the occasional drink or none at all.

Medications and Drugs

Almost all drugs cross to the fetus to varying degrees. It has been shown that many drugs can have harmful effects on the developing embryo. Although these effects are more likely to occur during the first three months of pregnancy, when the fetal organs are in their most critical formative stages, various medications are also known to harm the fetus when taken later in pregnancy. Therefore, all drugs should be avoided during your pregnancy except as advised by your doctor. Under no circumstances should you take any medicines that may be in use by well-meaning friends or relatives, since various commonly used medications can all pose dangers to your baby when unwisely used.

Aspirin. There is no known risk of birth defects when

aspirin is taken in the first three months. However, aspirin does inhibit uterine contractions and can delay the onset of labor as well as prolong labor. Aspirin also inhibits platelet function, which contributes to increased risk of bleeding. Thus if a mild drug for pain is necessary, acetaminophen (Tylenol or Datril) is preferred in pregnancy.

Low doses of aspirin (one baby aspirin daily) may help prevent preeclampsia, or pregnancy-induced high blood pressure, and research is active in this area. Ask your doctor about this if you have a history of this problem.

Antibiotics. Most antibiotics are safe when used appropriately. An exception is tetracycline, which causes discoloration of the infant's baby teeth if the drug is taken from the middle of pregnancy onward, and therefore alternative antibiotics are usually recommended. Penicillin and erythromycin are safe to use when necessary.

6

PREGNANCY AND
WEIGHT GAIN

The desirability of restricting *excessive* weight gain in pregnancy was stressed in the previous chapter. Many expectant mothers gain excessively despite attempts to eliminate rich desserts and snacks between meals. If your weight gain during the fourth month and after (see Figure 7, page 83) is around a pound a week (that is, at a rate that will not yield a total gain of more than twenty five to thirty pounds), it is unnecessary for you to read this chapter. If, however, the scales show a weekly increase in excess of one pound, so that you face a total gain of more than thirty pounds, it will repay you to study these next few pages carefully. In addition to the several advantages that you will now derive from better dietary management (as stressed on pages 80–81), there are even more important benefits to be gained from a general familiarity with this subject. As all life insurance statistics attest, obesity is a menace to the well-being and longevity of every man and woman; and obesity, with rare exceptions, is the result of faulty dietary habits. Accordingly, the general principles set forth in the Eight Steps below, although designed for your help in pregnancy, may well be remembered over the years to the advantage of every member of your family.

A Few Reminders

Physical activity is as much a part of the weight picture as is calorie intake; everything we do uses up energy, which is resupplied by energy derived from what we eat and drink. If oversupplied, this energy is stored in the body in the form of fat. Thus, if by the middle of the fourth month you are gaining more than a pound a week, and then start a regular exercise program without increasing your calorie intake, the *rate of gain* should decrease because you are using up more calories than before but not increasing the resupply level. If the extra demand for calories runs higher than the amount you are providing, the body draws on the stored fat for the energy it needs.

This factor and many others, including those of your personal body chemistry and your weight patterns before pregnancy, make it important for you to discuss any weight control program with your doctor. But assuming the doctor's approval, an appropriate exercise program with no calorie increase (perhaps even a decrease) is a fine way to help reduce extra weight gain.

Needless to say, maintaining adequate nutrition is the first requirement of any food plan, including a plan intended to reduce calorie intake. The Eight Steps are based on the principles in chapter 4 — to use all four food groups in your daily menus, maintain variety within the groups and supply vitamin and mineral as well as protein requirements. Unless so advised by your doctor, *do not consider any plan that involves quick weight loss* or abandon these nutritional principles even temporarily.

If you are gaining more than a pound a week, adjust the terms in the Eight Steps to match your own situation (for "milk" read "nonfat milk" and so on), and pay particular attention to the first four steps.

You may find that joining with a group of people with the same problem appeals to you as a help in actually carrying out your program for reducing excessive weight gain. Most physicians approve of such group arrangements when they are responsibly organized and conducted.

The Eight Steps in Weight Control

Step 1: Counting Calories

If you are not already familiar with the amazing fattening potential of certain common food items often regarded as mere snacks or little extras, take time to really look at the question now. Remember especially that: (1) Extra fat represents (among other factors) stored food energy. (2) Many higher-calorie foods supply important nutritional elements, for example, vegetable oils, at 125 calories per tablespoon, are a major source of vitamin E. (3) Others supply next to nothing except calories, with nutrients (if any) that can be found elsewhere in foods with a far smaller load of accompanying calories.

These last foods tend to fall in the category of "mere snacks" or "little extras" between meals or at bedtime, and thus constitute one of the most common causes of excessive weight gain. A one-ounce chocolate bar averages 145 calories (with almonds 150), a one-and-a-half-ounce cocktail or highball around 100. A doughnut (without icing) plus a cup of hot chocolate contain more than 350 calories, while one glass of malted milk contains 245. Pie à la mode approximates 400 calories. When it is recalled (see page 59) that 2,300 to 2,400 calories per day is generally recognized as a satisfactory allowance for pregnancy, it is plain that these items loom tremendously large in relation to the whole calorie allotment. If you are gaining excessively, they are best eliminated. To take the place of these snacks — or others like them — when you are hungry between meals try taking some of your daily milk allotment with a low-calorie raw vegetable snack such as carrot or celery sticks, a few leaves of salad greens, strips of green pepper, or radishes. Or enjoy the natural sweetness of an orange or orange juice — an eight-ounce glass contributes significant minerals and vitamins for 120 calories, including a minimum requirement of vitamin C for the day.

A list of some of the more common fattening foods is given at the end of the chapter (page 104). If you have trouble with extra weight, glance through this list and note the appalling number of calories in the snack type of food. Desserts also should be noted particularly — not overlooking what happens when you add ice cream to pie, fudge sauce to ice cream, and so on.

Step 2: Preparation of Foods

Remember that the way food is prepared may affect its calorie count or fattening value almost as much as the character of the food itself. Failure to heed this aspect has resulted in weight gain for many people on diets that should cause them, theoretically at least, to lose. Thus, in a typical day's menu as shown at the end of the chapter (pages 106–110), the calories may range from 2,300 to 3,400 depending on the ingredients used in the recipe, the cooking method, and of course the particular type of fruit, meat, and other items chosen. Perhaps the simplest example of the way food preparation affects the number of calories is to be found in frying. Although a poached or boiled egg has about 80 calories and is so calculated in dietary lists, the calories jump to around 100 for a fried egg because of the fat it absorbs in cooking. A level tablespoon of fat, let it be emphasized, yields 100 to 125 calories. Furthermore, many foods are coated with high-calorie batters, flour, or crumbs before frying, and this adds greatly to their caloric value. In regard to soups and desserts, it is common knowledge that those made with milk are much lower in calories than those made with cream, and that those made with skim or nonfat milk are still lower. When flour or crumbs are used in addition to milk or cream, as in scalloped or au gratin dishes, the calories increase even more, and in general for this group of foods, the smoother and more delicious the taste, unfortunately, the higher the caloric value.

The intrinsic caloric value of foods of the same type varies widely. Fruits show considerable variation according to their degree of sweetness. Canned fruit may be very high because of the sugar in the syrup. Meats vary also, those with a high fat content being high in calories. As an example of the latter, an average serving of linked country sausage is around 250 calories.

In summary, Step 2 consists of familiarizing yourself with the caloric effects of various ways of preparing or serving foods — and acting on them. The chief points are as follows: (1) Fried foods invariably possess a high caloric content, and should be curtailed or eliminated altogether. (2) Sugar adds calories at the rate of 15 per teaspoon. (3) Milk, preferably nonfat, should be used instead of cream in preparing soups, desserts, and other dishes. (4) Lean rather than fatty meats should be chosen, and fresh fruit rather than canned. (If canned fruits are used, choose those packed in juice rather than syrup.)

Step 3: Average Servings

Make certain that the size of servings eaten is not excessive, and that only one serving is taken — except, of course, for low-calorie vegetables. The standard household measuring cup (eight fluid ounces, which equals sixteen tablespoons) is a reference standard in describing amounts of food, as you will note in the tables in the appendixes. (See Appendix II for further measurements.)

Average servings of some of the more common foods are considered to be about:

Breakfast cereals (cooked or dry)	¾ to 1 cup
Potatoes, corn, lima beans, peas, macaroni, etc. (cooked)	½ cup
Other cooked vegetables	½ cup
Butter or margarine	1 pat (1 inch square, ⅓ inch thick)
Desserts such as puddings, custards, ice cream, gelatin desserts, etc.	½ cup

Step 4: 2,300-Calorie Diet

Having reviewed Steps 1, 2, and 3, you are now prepared to look again at the typical day's menus on page 110, and to ask yourself whether the diet you have been following is of the order of 2,300 calories, as shown in the

Pregnancy and Weight Gain

first figure in the calorie column, or whether, through disregard of the above steps, the menu has been calorically
expanded so that it approaches the second figure in the
column. To summarize the first three steps: Nothing is to
be eaten between meals (even if you spread the usual three
meals a day into five or six smaller meals) except part of
your milk or citrus fruit allotment or a low-calorie raw
vegetable snack. Foods are to be selected and prepared in a
way that will result in lower rather than higher numbers of
calories. Servings are to be "average" as defined in Step 3,
with no seconds except for low-calorie vegetables.

If these steps are followed conscientiously, the majority
of expectant mothers who have been troubled by excessive
weight gain will be able to reduce the gain to a pound a
week on this 2,300-calorie diet. The difficulty is that many
people who think they are following such a diet are actually exceeding it through nibbles between meals, or injudi-
cious selection and preparation of foods, or overlarge or
additional servings. Step 4, then, is a thorough review of
your experience so far, and revision as needed to make the
daily food plan conform to Steps 1, 2, and 3.

Step 5: Nonfat Milk

But what if you belong to the small minority group in
whom undesirably large weight gain persists despite rigorous adherence to the above suggestions? The next step —
which you may have already taken, as noted earlier — is to
review the previously advised practice of substituting nonfat (skim) milk for whole milk in your food plan. This
immediately reduces the number of calories in the diet by
about 300 — no small sum. But be sure to continue taking
adequate milk every day. It provides more protein, minerals, and vitamins for fewer calories (and money) than any

101

other food; and nonfat milk has, of course, as much protein and mineral content (including calcium) as whole milk. The vitamin A content is drastically reduced, but commercial nonfat milk is generally fortified with vitamin A.

Step 6: Sugar Substitutes

This step is an easy one and, with Step 7, may well be taken along with Step 5. In Step 6, you use a sugar substitute in coffee or tea. For every level teaspoon of sugar previously in the diet, 15 calories will be deleted — and every little bit helps.

Saccharin carries warnings that it may be hazardous to your health, and is best avoided in pregnancy. As there have been few studies of aspartame (NutraSweet, Equal) ingestion in pregnancy, it would seem appropriate to limit intake to a small amount of NutraSweet-containing foods per day, as alternative drinks such as club soda are clearly without risk. However, there are no theoretical reasons to believe it would be harmful, unless the mother had unrecognized PKU. For women who abhor the idea of drinking plain club soda (or salt-free seltzer), adding a splash of a favorite fruit juice will add flavor without many calories.

Step 7: Salt

Do not add *excessive* salt to foods either in cooking or at the table. As already mentioned (page 79), there is a relationship between the amount of salt eaten and the amount of water retained by the body; and it is quite possible, therefore, that a reduction in excessive sodium and chloride (salt) intake will release superfluous body water and cause a substantial weight loss. Nowadays most physicians advise the expectant mother to use the level of sodium intake she prefers, as long as it is not excessive.

Step 8: Cereals and Desserts

If excessive weight gain still persists, use unsweetened breakfast cereal, and for dessert use only fresh fruits, sweetened if necessary with a sugar substitute. This should delete between 200 and 300 calories and bring the total caloric intake nearer the norm for pregnancy.

It should be remembered that these steps are ongoing suggestions, to be reviewed as necessary with your doctor on your regular periodic visits, when you will be weighed and your progress evaluated. Steps to be implemented will be reflected also in the information on the weight grid (page 83) as your pregnancy advances.

It is rare for expectant mothers, even though they have rather sedentary habits, to gain excessively if they are actually, day in and day out, on a 2,200-calorie diet. If, however, you have followed conscientiously the steps listed above and are still gaining more than you should, note carefully the following. *Do not attempt, on the basis of instructions or facts given in this book or in any other book or article, to reduce your calorie intake to a level below that reached by these steps.* If these measures do not yield the desired result, you should be under the immediate and personal dietary supervision of either your physician or a nutritional consultant approved by your physician. Above all, do not curtail the basic food group recommendations for daily servings (pages 61–77). It may possibly be that your physician or nutritional consultant will even suggest some cutbacks here, but do not take this responsibility yourself or attempt in any other way to be your own dietitian at levels under 2,200 calories.

TABLE 1
Typical Foods for Consideration
in Step 1 (page 97)
(See also Appendix III)

Food and quantity	Number of calories
Corn chips, ¼ cup	60
Potato chips, 10 chips, 1¾ × 2½ inches	115
Pretzel, thin, twisted, 1	25
Root beer, 12 ounces	150
Soda, fruit flavored, 8 ounces	115
Beer, 12 ounces	150
Liqueur, 100 proof, 1½ ounces	125
Whiskey, gin, rum, vodka, 80 proof, 1½ ounces	95
Wine, table, 3½ ounces	85
Chocolate bar, 1 ounce	145
With almonds	150
Mints, 1 ounce (3 1½ inch mints)	105
Brownie, with nuts, 1¾ inches square, ⅞ inch thick	90
Cake, plain, un-iced, 3 × 3 × 2 inch piece	315
Cookie, chocolate chip, 2⅓ inches across, ½ inch thick	50
Fudge sauce, 1 tablespoon	60
Ice cream, plain, about 10 percent fat, ½ cup	130
Jelly or marmalade, 1 tablespoon	50

Table 1 (continued)

Food and quantity	Number of calories
Pie, apple, ⅛ of 9 inch pie	300
Sugar, 1 teaspoon	15
Danish pastry, plain, 4½ inches diameter	275
Doughnut, raised (yeast), 3¾ inches diameter	175
Waffle, 7 inch	210
Hot chocolate, 1 cup (8 ounces)	215
Malted milk, 1 cup (8 ounces)	245
Whipped cream (from heavy cream), about 2 tablespoons	55
White sauce, medium (1 cup milk, 2 tablespoons each of fat and flour), ½ cup	200
Butter or margarine, 1 pat (1 inch square, ⅓ inch thick)	35
Mayonnaise, 1 tablespoon	100
Vegetable shortening, 1 tablespoon	110
Bologna, 2 very thin slices, 4½ inches diameter (2 ounces)	170
French fries, fresh, 3½ × ¼ inch, 10 pieces	215
Hamburger, 2 ounce patty with roll	280
Pizza, plain cheese, 5½ inch section of 13¾ inch round	155
Sausage, link, 4 sausages, each 4 inches long (uncooked, 4 ounces)	250

TABLE 2
A Typical Day's Menu

The calorie total in this type of menu can range from 2,300 to upwards of 3,000, depending on the type of food selected, the methods of cooking and serving (see page 98), and the quantity eaten. The recommended total for a pregnant woman is 2,300 to 2,400 calories.

Breakfast

Item	Calories	Change or addition	Plus calories
Grapefruit half, pink	50	Sugar, 1 teaspoon	15
Cornflakes, ⅔ cup	65	Sugar-coated cornflakes, ⅔ cup (110)	45
Milk, ½ cup	80		
Egg, poached	80	Egg, fried (100)	20
Toast, 2 slices* whole-wheat	120		
Margarine or butter, 1 pat†	35		
Jelly or marmalade, 1 tablespoon	50		

* Eighteen slices to a 1-pound loaf.
† Pat of margarine or butter is 1 inch square and ⅓ inch thick.

Breakfast (continued)

Item	Calories	Change or addition	Plus calories
Beverage (coffee, tea, etc.)	—	Sugar, 1 teaspoon	15
		Coffee cream, 1 tablespoon	30
		Doughnut	165
Total calories	480	Added calories	290
		Expanded total	770

Lunch

Beef bouillon, 1 cup, with lemon wedge	30	Butter crackers, 3	45
Salmon cheese loaf	285	White sauce, 3 tablespoons	75
Green peas, ½ cup (65) with ½ teaspoon margarine or butter (15)	80		
Small tomato sliced (20), with ½ tablespoon mixed salad oil, lemon juice, seasonings (60)	80		

Lunch (continued)

Item	Calories	Change or addition	Plus calories
Whole-wheat roll (105) with 1 pat margarine or butter (35)	140		
Fruit: for example, mixed blueberries and peaches, ½ cup	40	Instead of fruit and cookies: blueberry pie, ⅛ of 9-inch pie (285)	180
Honey (about 1 teaspoon) and lemon juice over the fruit	25		
Vanilla wafers, 1¼ inch diameter, 2	40		
Total calories	720	Added calories	300
		Expanded total	1020

Dinner

Pot roast, 4 ounces	325		
Gravy, 2 tablespoons	35	More gravy (about a tablespoon)	20
Vegetables: ⅓ cup onions (20)			

Dinner (continued)

Item	Calories	Change or addition	Plus calories
⅓ cup diced carrots (15), ½ cup diced potatoes (65)	100		
		Whole-wheat roll (105) and 1 pat butter (35)	140
Salad of cucumber, celery, green pepper, and radish, with lettuce (15), with ½ tablespoon mixed salad oil, vinegar, seasonings (60)	75		
Apple snow, about ½ cup, with 2 tablespoons custard sauce	55		
Thin oatmeal cookies, 2	80	Instead of cookies: plain cake, 2 × 2 × 2 inches (1/16 of 8-inch square cake) (140)	60
Total calories	670	*Added calories*	220
		Expanded total	890

Other

Item	Calories	Change or addition	Plus calories
Nonfat milk, 2½ cups (1½ cups milk used in menus)	225	Whole milk, 2½ cups (400)	175
Miscellaneous (juices, fruit or vegetable snacks)	205	Plus 10 potato chips	115
Total calories	430	*Added calories*	290
		Expanded total	720

Total Calories for the Day

	Total calories	+ Additions =	Total with extras
Breakfast	480	290	770
Lunch	720	300	1020
Dinner	670	220	890
Other	430	290	720
Day's total	2300	1100	3400

NOTE: This sample menu does not include beverages other than at breakfast and the daily milk allowance.

7

COMMON DISCOMFORTS
AND THEIR TREATMENT

Nausea

It is common knowledge that the early weeks of pregnancy are frequently associated with some degree of nausea. In mapping out a regimen to correct this tendency it is helpful to recall certain factors that predispose to nausea in the nonpregnant person, because these same factors are commonly responsible for the nausea expectant mothers experience. Strong odors or fumes, and spicy or greasy foods may aggravate the tendency to be nauseated. In addition, certain hormone changes that occur early in pregnancy undoubtedly contribute to the occurrence of nausea in some women. Do not anticipate being nauseated simply because "morning sickness" is an old tradition of pregnancy, as more than a third of all pregnant women escape it altogether.

A second circumstance that can cause nausea in the pregnant and nonpregnant alike is an empty stomach. Thus, many patients note that the stomach is more unsettled in the morning before breakfast. This is a very important fact to bear in mind, for it is the basis of the most effective treatment of the condition; namely, a regimen of

111

small meals taken at frequent intervals so that the stomach, as far as is possible, may never become empty. Since dry food is most easily retained, crackers and toast should be given a prominent place in the dietary program, as the following plan exemplifies:

1. Before going to bed, place two or more crackers and perhaps some juice on a table beside the bed. Upon awakening, eat the crackers without raising the head from the pillow; then remain lying down for a number of minutes.

2. A nourishing but not heavy breakfast, let us say brown cereal and milk, toast, and coffee. Butter or margarine should not be used on the toast; substitute marmalade, jelly, or honey.

3. 10:30 A.M. Crackers or toast with a glass of juice or nonfat (or low-fat) milk, or a cup of hot chocolate, tea, or hot malted milk.

4. Lunch: Vegetable soup with crackers; rice; a green vegetable or a fruit salad; bread or rolls.

5. 4 P.M. Crackers or toast with a glass of orange juice, grapefruit juice, or lemonade.

6. Dinner: Lean meat; green vegetable; baked, boiled, or mashed potatoes; tomato and lettuce salad; dessert.

7. Before going to bed, crackers or toast with a glass of juice or nonfat (or low-fat) milk, or a piece of cheese, or a cup of hot chocolate, tea, or hot malted milk. Chocolate, tea, and coffee all contain caffeine, which should of course be used in moderation, especially at bedtime.

It must be understood that this diet is only a temporary makeshift until the nausea subsides. As soon as it has definitely passed, the menu should be greatly augmented and diversified, as recommended in the previous chapter.

A third cause of nausea in both the pregnant and the

nonpregnant is found in fried and greasy foods, and these, together with butter and margarine, must be deleted from the diet. Likewise, cabbage, cauliflower, and spinach are often upsetting. Although water may prove to be troublesome, every effort should be made to consume the equivalent of six glasses of fluid a day in some form, such as hot chocolate, milk, soups, or ginger ale.

Relief from nausea is often obtained by lying down and it is a good plan to do this whenever the sensation comes on. Some women, indeed, find that the discomfort can be forestalled altogether by lying down regularly for twenty minutes immediately after each meal. The beneficial effect of the horizontal position is often enhanced by placing an ice bag or a towel wrung out in cold water over the region of the stomach.

In the vast majority of cases the measures outlined above, if followed meticulously, will put an end to the nausea. If they do not — particularly if the condition is associated with actual vomiting — the condition should be reported to your doctor, and medications may be prescribed. Taking ten to twenty-five milligrams of Vitamin B_6 three times a day may also be helpful.

Heartburn

Heartburn is a burning sensation in the upper abdomen or lower part of the chest, sometimes associated with the belching of small amounts of bitter fluid. It has nothing to do with the heart, but involves regurgitation of acidic juice from the stomach into the esophagus and is actually a mild form of indigestion. In view of this fact, the first step in the treatment of the condition should be a careful survey of

113

one's dietary habits to make sure that rich and indigestible foods are omitted and that overeating and hurried eating are avoided. Common compounds such as Maalox or Gelusil that may be purchased over the counter are often helpful but should not be overused. Liquid antacids are more effective than tablets. Some people seem to be relieved by chewing gum. Ask your physician about acceptable medications. *Do not* take baking soda (sodium bicarbonate), as it does not effectively coat the esophagus but is absorbed readily.

Flatulence

Distention of the stomach and intestines with gas, a condition known as flatulence, may accompany heartburn or appear independently. In pregnancy it is usually caused by the hormonal affects of pregnancy on the bowel and by bacterial action in the intestines. In addition, the pressure of the enlarged uterus hinders the intestinal contents from moving along as rapidly as usual. Because of this, the primary consideration in the treatment of flatulence is regular evacuation of the bowels. Another important preventive measure is to chew all solid food very slowly and thoroughly. At the same time, care should be taken to avoid gas-producing foods such as beans, parsnips, corn, onions, cabbage, fried foods, and sweet desserts.

Constipation

Many women who have always been quite regular become constipated in pregnancy because of the pressure of the enlarged uterus on the lower intestine, plus the relaxing effect of pregnancy hormones on the muscle tissues of the bowel. Iron tablets may aggravate the condition. Regular bowel movements may be expedited by a few simple measures such as the following:

1. Upon arising drink a glass or two of cold water. While hot water may be substituted if desired, cold has a more stimulating effect on the digestive tract. A few drops of lemon juice may make the drink more refreshing.

2. Eat a coarse cereal such as oatmeal or bran for breakfast. Marmalade with breakfast is beneficial, since its juices are laxative and the pieces of hard orange skin act as a mechanical stimulus to the bowel.

3. Eat some fruit at night before going to bed. Fruits are helpful not only in adding bulk to the stool, but also because their juices contain various acids, sugars, and salts that are laxative. Certain fruits, of course, are particularly effective, notably prunes, figs, raisins, dates, and apples. Prunes enjoy a well-deserved reputation as a laxative agent, and a small quantity of prune juice at night may be all that is necessary.

4. Eat plenty of green vegetables, both raw and cooked. These add so-called roughage to the stool and thereby stimulate the eliminative action of the intestines. Whole-wheat bread has the same tendency and should be used instead of white bread.

5. Make a habit of going to the toilet at a regular time, preferably after breakfast.

6. Stool softeners, such as Colace (docusate) or Metamucil soften the stool without a laxative effect, and counteract the effect of iron tablets, which harden the stool. They may be taken one to three times a day, as

necessary. Most physicians have no objection to the expectant mother's taking milk of magnesia, a tablespoonful at bedtime, but she should employ no other laxative without her doctor's advice.

Hemorrhoids (Piles)

These are formed by enlarged and dilated veins at the opening of the rectum. Pregnancy contributes to their development because the growing uterus tends to obstruct the blood flow in the region of the rectum and thus interferes with the emptying of the veins. Pregnancy alone, however, does not actually produce hemorrhoids unless constipation is present, because the two underlying causes are hard stools and straining at stool. Under these circumstances the veins become enlarged, stretched, and painful; not infrequently the condition is associated with itching and slight bleeding. It is only common sense, therefore, that the first step in the treatment of the hemorrhoids is correction of constipation.

Pending advice from your physician, painful hemorrhoids are best treated by sitz baths or tub baths, but water temperature should not exceed 39° Celsius (102° Fahrenheit). If the hemorrhoids are extruded, they can be replaced with the finger. Ointments, cold cream, or petroleum jelly are often soothing.

Varicose Veins

Just as the enlarged uterus tends to obstruct blood flow from the rectal region, so it may likewise interfere with blood flow from the lower extremities and give rise to swollen veins in the legs. Varicose veins are not likely to develop in the course of a first pregnancy, but may be very annoying in women who have previously had children. Tight girdles and stockings aggravate any tendency in this direction and should not be used. The treatment is of two kinds. In the first place, every opportunity should be taken to elevate the legs on a pillow so that the heel is slightly higher than the hip. It is even more effective to lie down on the left side, taking the weight of the pregnancy off the veins coming from the legs. The more this is done at odd times in the day and evening, the better. Second, if this simple postural treatment is insufficient, elastic (support) stockings or panty hose should be worn. The stockings should be put on in the morning so that support is given to the veins when they are well emptied from the night's elevation of the legs.

Muscular Cramps

During the later weeks of pregnancy, muscular cramps in the back and thighs are a common source of discomfort. The enlarged, protruding uterus calls for a backward tilt of the torso if equilibrium is to be maintained — a posture that imposes a constant strain on the back and thigh muscles whenever you are on your feet. Appropriate exercise can help strengthen these muscles. Adequate amounts of rest are the best preventive. A well-fitting maternity girdle and moderately low heels are also beneficial. A considerable degree of immediate relief may be obtained by massage of the group of muscles involved. In this connection it is interesting to recall that liniments by the carload have been sold by patent medicine companies with the claim that they are specific for this very trouble. They are of no value, since it is the massage employed in rubbing the liniment in that is soothing, not any magic drug in the liniment. Shooting pains down the legs are sometimes caused by pressure of the baby's head on certain nerves. If pains of this type are severe, it may be worthwhile to try sitting or lying in a different position for a few minutes.

Fainting

Dizzy spells and actual fainting attacks are experienced by a few women, particularly during the first half of pregnancy. These may be related to a decrease in blood flow from the legs into the circulation, due to the obstruction from the pregnancy. Avoid prolonged standing, and exercise the calves to keep the circulation going. Also avoid lying flat on your back — a side tilt will keep the pressure of the uterus off the veins.

Shortness of Breath

As a result of the upward pressure of the enlarged uterus against the lungs, shortness of breath is common during the last two months. In first pregnancies, decided relief is usually experienced a week or two before delivery because the baby's head sinks into the pelvis, thereby giving more room above. If shortness of breath interferes with sleep, the head and shoulders should be comfortably propped up with several pillows so that a semi-sitting posture is assumed. Almost invariably this relieves shortness of breath to the extent that a restful night's sleep may be had. In general, avoidance of the supine position helps alleviate the problem. Although some shortness of breath is perfectly normal in the later weeks of pregnancy, it should be reported to your physician if it reaches such a degree that you cannot climb a flight of stairs without discomfort.

Insomnia

Although the early part of pregnancy is often accompanied by an overpowering desire to sleep, the later weeks are sometimes associated with insomnia. Many factors contribute to this, including movements of the baby, shortness of breath, and muscular cramps — to say nothing of thoughts about the coming infant. A short walk in the open air before bedtime, followed by a warm bath or shower and a glass of milk, will often help. You may sleep in any position in which you are comfortable, for there is no possibility of "compressing" the baby; a heating pad or hot water bag at the feet or an extra pillow under the head may help.

Round Ligament Pain

Occasionally there will be sharp pains in the groin, more frequently on the right than on the left, associated with movement. This is due to a spasm in the muscle in the so-called round ligament, which is the ligament that supports the uterus on each side in the front. The pain may be helped by applying local heat such as with a hot water bottle or heating pad. Sometimes you may wake up at night with this pain after having suddenly rolled over in your sleep without realizing it. During the daytime, modification of activity with gradual rising and sitting down and avoidance of sudden movement will decrease problems with this type of pain. Medications are rarely necessary.

Backache

Backache can be prevented to a large degree by avoiding excessive weight gain. Exercises to strengthen back muscles can also be helpful. Posture is important and sensible shoes should be worn, not high heels.

Vaginal Discharge

Moderate vaginal discharge is common in the later part of pregnancy because of seepage of fluids from the congested vagina and neck of the uterus. (Incidentally, tampons should not be used in pregnancy.) The discharge is ordinarily pale yellow in color and thin. If thick in consistency or very profuse, or if associated with itching, it should be reported to the physician. In most cases external cleansing with warm water is all that is necessary. As we have already emphasized, douches must not be taken unless detailed instructions are received from your doctor.

If there is sudden leakage of watery fluid, even in small quantities, it should be reported to the physician as occasionally it may represent a break in the bag of waters.

8

DANGER SIGNALS

I f you have ever grown flowers, you will recall that even
in the best-kept garden an occasional sprout will show
signs of blight, evidence that something is interfering with
the normal process of plant reproduction. You will also
realize that if this plant is properly sprayed at the very first
signs of the fungus infection, the disease is eradicated and
the sprout develops normally; whereas if the blight is allowed to progress untreated, havoc may result. Now let us
suppose that we have an expert horticulturist in charge of
our hypothetical garden, one who diligently and at frequent intervals inspects each sprout, and at the very first
sign of trouble institutes with professional skill the type of
treatment long experience has shown to be best. Surely,
then, there would be no cause to worry about our flowers!
In human reproduction the situation is similar, for here
also things sometimes go wrong, but here, likewise, early
recognition by a trained observer, together with intelligent
treatment, usually results in cure. Very often the expectant
mother is not aware of these disturbances and in the early
stages of certain common complications may feel quite
well. Only the physician's careful examination can detect
the beginning of a disturbance, and only by seeing her

doctor regularly can the expectant mother be certain that deviations from the normal will be detected at their onset and as quickly corrected.

Sometimes, between visits to her doctor, the expectant mother may notice a change in her condition that merits reporting to the physician at once. More often than not, the change does not turn out to indicate trouble; nevertheless, the physician should be notified without delay so that the situation may be examined and treated if necessary.

Symptoms That Demand Immediate Report to the Physician

1. VAGINAL BLEEDING, NO MATTER HOW SLIGHT.
2. SWELLING OF THE FACE OR FINGERS.
3. SEVERE, CONTINUOUS HEADACHE.
4. DIMNESS OR BLURRING OF VISION.
5. PAIN IN THE ABDOMEN, OR MENSTRUAL-LIKE CRAMPS.
6. PERSISTENT VOMITING.
7. CHILLS AND FEVER.
8. SUDDEN ESCAPE OF WATER FROM THE VAGINA.

Although these symptoms may sound formidable, their significance depends entirely on the circumstances under which they occur. Even the development of several of them may be quite normal and not necessarily a cause for concern. For instance, the onset of normal labor is often heralded by a very slight amount of bleeding, recurrent pain in the abdomen, and a discharge of water from the vagina. Usually, however, these symptoms deserve particular attention because they often constitute warnings of the most common complications of pregnancy: namely, ectopic pregnancy, miscarriage, toxemia, urinary tract infection, placenta previa, and premature separation of the placenta. It is true that there are other complications of pregnancy, but they are so rare that the average woman's chance of experiencing any one of them is less than one in one hundred. In view of this, let us limit our discussion to these more common conditions.

Ectopic Pregnancy

Vaginal bleeding is sometimes associated with ectopic pregnancy. This is a pregnancy that is growing outside the uterus, most commonly in one of the two tubes. It occurs when the egg, after fertilization by the sperm, fails to properly migrate into the uterine cavity and attach itself and grow there, as shown in Figure 2. Ectopic pregnancies usually cause internal bleeding and pain requiring surgery. They commonly do not progress beyond the first few gestational weeks.

Implantation Bleeding

It should be noted that in 20 to 30 percent of patients, there may be slight bleeding when the fertilized egg burrows into the uterine lining and implants itself (see page 24). This "implantation bleeding" is a normal phenomenon and usually occurs before or near the time of the first missed menstrual period.

Miscarriage

In general use, the word *miscarriage* means the birth of a fetus before it is sufficiently developed to live outside the mother's body; that is, usually before the twenty-fourth week of pregnancy. Doctors, however, ordinarily refer to this same occurrence not as a miscarriage but as an abortion. Thus the word *abortion* in medical terminology and the word *miscarriage* in general use are somewhat synonymous. Accordingly, if your doctor inquires if you have ever had an abortion, the question is simply whether you have ever had a pregnancy that terminated in the early months. For medical purposes, it is very important that you give full details of any such occurrence. When physicians wish to indicate that the event was not a spontaneous abortion but was brought on intentionally, they speak of a "therapeutic" or "legal" abortion, meaning that it was performed by a physician for reasons within the law.

Miscarriages are very common; reliable estimates show that at least one pregnancy in every ten terminates of its own accord in this manner. Most miscarriages occur during the second and third months; thereafter the likelihood of the accident is decidedly less. What causes all these miscarriages — so tragic and shattering to so many women? Is nature actually as cruel as these figures suggest? If we review the situation with some perspective and with full fairness to all concerned, we must arrive at the inevitable conclusion that most of these miscarriages, far from being tragedies, are blessings in disguise, for they are nature's kind way of extinguishing an imperfect embryo. This is particularly true of very early miscarriages. Indeed, careful microscopic study of the material passed in the first two months shows that in 80 percent of these embryos some defect is present that is either incompatible with life or would result in a grossly deformed child. The incidence of abnormalities in embryos passed after the second month is somewhat lower, but not less than 50 percent. Some authorities believe that 80 percent of all miscarriages are ascribable to abnormalities in the embryo. Whether the problem derives from the female or male cell is usually difficult, if not impossible, to say. Miscarriages of this sort are obviously unpreventable, and although bitterly disappointing to the parents, they serve in the long run a useful purpose.

Since imperfectly formed embryos are almost always aborted early in pregnancy, there is much less likelihood of a full-term child's being defective. Not a few parents worry about this possibility as the time of delivery approaches, but when a woman is in the second half of pregnancy, the chances are fifty to one that the child will be born without any abnormalities.

Although many miscarriages are caused by factors other than defects in the embryo, little is known about these causes. In certain cases the uterus may be abnormally shaped, either since birth or as a result of the presence of fibroids, and this condition may very occasionally cause the accident. A visit to the physician before the next pregnancy can result in detection and correction of the abnormality and consequently a better outlook. Many women blame miscarriage on injury of one type or another, or excessive activity. There is great variation in this respect; in some women the pregnancy may go blithely on despite falls from second-story windows and automobile accidents so severe as to fracture the hip bone; in others a trivial fall or just overfatigue seems to be associated with miscarriage which may have been destined to occur anyhow. Since there is no way of foretelling who is susceptible to the accident and who is not, it would seem prudent for every expectant mother to follow the dictates of common sense and avoid lifting heavy weights and any form of activity than involves jolting.

• The first symptom of possible miscarriage is usually

bleeding. In some cases this begins as a little irregular spotting, followed in a day or two by a moderate discharge of blood that simulates a menstrual period; this may persist for several days before the onset of pain and increased bleeding denote the beginning of the process by which the pregnancy tissue is expelled. In other cases the bleeding may be profuse from the start and accompanied by recurrent cramplike pains, similar to those experienced sometimes during menstruation. Occasionally, pain is the first symptom of miscarriage, but in most cases it is preceded by bleeding.

At the first sign of bleeding — even the slightest spotting — the expectant mother should notify her doctor. Medical observation may reveal that there is simply a threatened miscarriage. Studies have shown that as many as 18 percent of normal pregnancies may have some bleeding in the early months without problems in later months or subsequent delivery of an abnormal infant. In other instances, however, the bleeding and the pain increase, and the tissue is expelled. If it is passed completely, no treatment may be necessary and the pregnancy terminates spontaneously. It frequently happens, however, that only part of the material is passed. In that event, depending on the amount of bleeding and other factors, it often becomes necessary for the doctor to remove the remainder. This procedure requires only a few minutes, and is not a serious operation. It is called a curettage, or cleaning of the lining of the womb with a spoonlike instrument, and is often done with local anesthesia. Since the treatment of any case of miscarriage depends in large measure on the completeness of the expulsion, it is extremely important that all material passed, including blood clots, be saved for the doctor to examine.

Danger Signals

Miscarriages that start of their own accord and receive proper treatment are rarely serious as far as the mother's physical welfare is concerned. Danger is very real, however, in self-dosing or other attempts to provoke the process intentionally. The results, all too often, are unbelievably tragic. Accustomed though we may be in this age of machinery, science, and "free thought" to disregard natural phenomena, pregnancy is one process of nature that it is best to treat with the utmost respect.

Some patients are under the impression that some drugs, such as castor oil, quinine, or other compounds, can produce a desired abortion. However, at the present writing there is no drug available for general use that will regularly produce miscarriage in the human being, whether given by mouth or by injection.

Preeclampsia (Toxemia)

During the latter part of pregnancy, for reasons that are unknown, the expectant mother occasionally manifests a group of signs and symptoms called toxemia, or preeclampsia. Although by derivation the word means "poison in the blood," no such poison has been demonstrated and it is generally agreed that this label is a misnomer. In the majority of cases the mother at first feels quite well, but medical examination shows an increase in the blood pressure; along with this, albumin may appear in the urine, indicating a kidney disturbance. The chief symptoms the mother herself may notice include: swelling of the face and fingers (are the eyes swollen in the morning? do rings become tight?), rapid gain in weight (bathroom scales are an asset throughout pregnancy), persistent headache unrelieved by the usual methods of treatment, and difficulty with the eyes such as blurring of vision. If the condition is

127

properly treated no harm comes to either mother or child, all these signs and symptoms disappearing entirely, as a rule, after the baby is born; but if it is neglected serious complications may ensue. It is important for the expectant mother to be aware of the toxemias of pregnancy for a number of reasons. She will understand, in the first place, why frequent blood pressure determinations are desirable during the later months. Second, in the event that a slight elevation of blood pressure should occur, she will appreciate the necessity for exact compliance with the doctor's instructions and will not minimize their importance merely because she "feels well"; paradoxically enough, a woman may feel well and yet be decidedly ill from toxemia. And finally, of course, she will realize the importance of communicating at once with her physician in case any of the symptoms mentioned above develop.

The treatment of toxemia of pregnancy depends very much upon the circumstances of each individual case. An important form of treatment in toxemia is rest. Frequently complete rest in bed is desirable; and to this end, physicians often suggest a few days' stay in the hospital, not only for the purpose of absolute rest but also in order for meticulous surveillance to be exercised over diet, weight control, blood pressure, and other essentials of treatment.

Urinary Tract Infection

The kidney pelvis, the funnellike portion of the kidney that conveys the urine from the kidney to the tube (ureter) leading to the bladder, is a common site of inflammation in pregnancy; the ureter itself may also be involved. This condition occurs about once in every fifty pregnancies; it is most likely to develop about the sixth month, but may make its appearance at any time in pregnancy. When you recall that the enlarged uterus presses backward against the ureter, it is easy to understand that the flow of urine through it could readily be impeded and that a certain degree of damming back of urine might result. When the flow of urine through the kidney pelvis and ureter is not brisk, stagnation is prone to ensue, with consequent inflammation. The characteristic symptoms are chills, fever, and pain in the upper back on one or the other side, but most frequently on the right. Urinary tract infection is rarely a serious condition, and usually responds readily to treatment. The most important thing for the expectant mother to know about urinary tract infection is that copious water drinking, six or eight glasses a day, by continually flushing out the kidneys, is a valuable preventive and renders the development of the condition most unlikely. Many doctors check the urine at the beginning of pregnancy for the presence of infection. Treatment then can prevent this kidney infection later.

Placenta Previa and Premature Separation of the Placenta
Vaginal bleeding during the third trimester of pregnancy may be associated with a condition called "placenta previa" ("placenta first"), in which the placenta is located over the uterine neck, the cervix. This condition blocks the delivery of the infant and the placenta detaches itself as the cervix dilates.

Late-pregnancy bleeding may also occur because of premature separation of the placenta, that is, when the placenta detaches before or during labor. Doctors call this "abruptio placentae." This premature separation of course decreases the supply of oxygen to the baby and may require immediate delivery. Bleeding under these circumstances is usually heavy and should be reported promptly to your doctor.

Preterm Labor Detection

If you have symptoms suggestive of labor well ahead of the due date, it is important to report these to the doctor. Warning signs include mild menstrual-like cramps, low backache, pelvic pressure, increased vaginal discharge, pink staining, and diarrhea. An examination will tell if the cervix is dilating or uterine contractions are occurring. If this is the case, medications can be used to stop preterm labor and prevent the baby from being born too soon.

Vaginal Leakage of Fluid

If the bag of waters leaks and fluid escapes from around the baby, this is a danger signal which should be reported promptly to the doctor. Many times labor will follow. However, if labor does not follow, an infection may result. The doctor may want to check you to determine if the discharge is indeed the amniotic fluid from around the baby or some other type of discharge. This can be done with a test called the nitrazine test, which checks the acidity of the fluid, and by looking at the fluid under the microscope. Amniotic fluid forms a ferning pattern which is not formed by other types of discharge.

Telephoning Your Doctor

If it becomes desirable to telephone your physician in order to report one or another symptom or make inquiries about it, bear in mind the following suggestions:

1. If the reason for the telephone call is vaginal bleeding

in pregnancy or a discharge of water from the vagina, be well informed about details. For instance, if the condition prompting the call is vaginal bleeding in pregnancy, how much blood is being passed? Is it mere spotting mixed with mucus? Is it as much as occurs on the first day of a menstrual period, or more, or less? Has there been any pain associated with the bleeding? If so, is it in the midline and cramplike in character or is it at one side of the abdomen, and if so, which side?

2. Talk to the doctor yourself if at all possible. To relay questions and answers back and forth through a third party is not only likely to result in a misleading story for the doctor, and garbled advice for you, but also trebles the time consumed by the call.

3. Provided the condition prompting the call is not one of the danger signals listed on page 122, call the physician's office during usual office hours.

4. Do not ask to speak to the doctor, but report the reason for your call to the secretary or nurse who answers the phone. The person serves as an assistant to the doctor and can deal with a good many matters completely to your satisfaction, or if necessary can consult the physician at a more convenient moment and call you back. If the reason for your call requires it, the nurse or secretary will make sure that the doctor either speaks to you at once or calls you back very shortly.

5. Have paper and pencil at hand when you make the call. Do not waste time looking for these articles after you have the physician on the phone.

6. Know the name, address, and telephone number of your pharmacy. The physician may want to telephone a prescription for you to that pharmacy, and obviously it will expedite matters if you can give the phone number.

9

PREPARATIONS FOR
THE BABY

The preparation of the baby's layette is naturally an important and enjoyable undertaking for every expectant mother. Fortunately for all concerned, the dictates of common sense have greatly simplified this problem in recent years, and the chief emphasis is on clothes that are comfortable for the baby and timesaving for the parents. They must be loose, of course, permitting complete freedom of motion. They should be light in weight and not too warm; the common tendency is to dress the baby too heavily, particularly in well-heated apartments — an error that often gives rise to skin irritation as well as to fretfulness. From everyone's point of view, the parents' and the baby's, the clothes should be easy to put on the baby and to take off again.

Often, the tendency is to buy too much rather than too little. The following three lists comprise all that you need to have ready, but they may be supplemented or modified according to individual taste.

The Layette

In general, all of the following materials should be of flame-retardant materials. Usually they will be so labeled.

6 *undershirts.* Cotton knit, 6-month size.
4 *cotton knit nightgowns.* These usually have a drawstring in the sleeves and at the bottom so that if the baby becomes uncovered during the night there will be no chilling of hands or feet.
3 *"stretch suits."* Made of various elasticized materials, such as terry cloth, and marketed under several trade names, these outfits are practical and comfortable.
2 *blanket-weight sleeping bags.* These take the place of blankets and are much more efficient in keeping the baby warm on cold nights.
2 *pairs bootees.* For occasional use.
2 *pairs socks.* For occasional use.
2 *sacques or sweaters.* These should open down the front.
1 *cap and coat or bunting.*
3 *dozen diapers.* For years no description of diapers was necessary, as there was only one kind, made of bird's eye, 22 × 22 inches. Today there are various choices. The old-fashioned bird's-eye diaper is still satisfactory if desired. There is also a very popular type, made of a fine porous webbing, that is prefolded according to lines woven in the material, making them easier to use and providing protection where most needed. There are also disposable diapers, to be thrown away after use, which are especially good for travel. Then, too, in most cities there are diaper services, which are extremely convenient; clean sterilized diapers are delivered regularly

and the soiled ones collected. But even if you employ a diaper service, it is prudent to have a dozen of your own on hand, disposable or otherwise, "just in case."

3 *pairs waterproof pants.* These can be of rubber, silk, or plastic; not necessary if you use disposable diapers.

4 *to 6 bibs.* For feedings and teething.

As for dresses, which used to be a standard item, a boy baby will never need one under ordinary circumstances, nor will a girl at this age unless you and her father wish to dress her up. Futhermore, you may be able to depend upon gifts supplying any deficiency.

Nursery Needs

1 *bed or basket.*

1 *mattress.*

6 *sheets.* Fitted crib sheets simplify bed making and provide a wrinkle-free surface.

1 *rubberized felt sheet* and 1 *rubberized felt pad.* These are preferred to rubber sheets for keeping the mattress dry.

6 *crib pads,* to be put under the baby. They should be quilted or made of Turkish toweling, and should measure about 18 × 18 inches.

1 *crib bumper pad,* to fit inside crib around sides, for protection of baby.

1 *woolen crib blanket.* This must be large enough to tuck under the baby's mattress.

4 *to 6 receiving blankets.*

1 *dressing table or bathinette.* This is invaluable for bathing, dressing, and changing the baby. Several folding types with plastic top, plastic bathtub, and pockets for acces-

sories are available at department stores. Check safety
factors thoroughly before buying; avoid sharp edges
and corners, inadequate catches that may cause col-
lapse, and so on.

The Baby's Tray

3 *nursing bottles* (8-ounce). More will be required if the
baby is bottle-fed. Presterilized disposable "inner bottles" possess certain advantages but are somewhat expensive. Your pediatrician may have suggestions in this
regard.
6 *nipples.*
1 *nipple jar.*
1 *bottle brush.*
3 *covered jars.* For cotton balls. (For cleansing around the
baby's ears and nostrils, use the corner of a wash cloth,
not so-called "swabs.")
Safety pins (large and small). A bar of soap makes an excellent "safety-pin cushion," since it lubricates the points
of the pins, making it easier to insert them into the diapers.
Absorbent cotton.
Soap.
Baby oil, lotion, and powder.
4 *washcloths* (knitted, smooth).
2 *hand towels* (knitted, smooth).
2 *bath towels* (knitted, smooth).

An additional item you will need is an *infant car seat.*
When you leave the hospital with your baby, it is the law
in many states that the baby be transported in an infant car

seat, rather than being held by you or another passenger. This is an important safety precaution, and applies as well to older children.

Questions regarding additional preparations and plans for the baby's early care should be brought to your doctor or to the pediatrician who will look after the baby. Most pediatricians welcome the opportunity to meet you and discuss these matters in advance of your delivery.

10

ALTERNATIVES AND METHODS OF CHILDBIRTH

Alternatives

Over the years there has been an increased emphasis on childbirth as an experience to be shared by both parents, and sometimes the whole family. This in turn has given rise to alternative locations and styles for giving birth, ranging from the traditional hospital delivery, to ABC's (Alternative Birthing Centers), to delivery at home. There can be advantages to some of these alternatives depending upon the supervision available and the training and information provided. You should discuss with your doctor the pros and cons of the alternatives available in your area.

Hospital Delivery

More than 90 percent of the births in the United States now take place in hospitals; hence, the problem of hospital versus home delivery is usually not much of a question. However, since there is some opinion in favor of home delivery, it would seem appropriate to review the advantages of hospital delivery.

Hospitalization for childbirth is a development of the

past five decades. In the early years of this century it was nearly impossible to persuade a respectable woman to enter a hospital for normal delivery, since only the derelicts of womankind and the destitute sought hospitalization for such a purpose. The present popularity of the hospital, then, has been achieved against great odds and can only mean that hospital care has proved its value to millions of satisfied mothers. It is often said that doctors are largely responsible for this change because of the great convenience it provides them. While this has doubtless been a factor, the change could not have been brought about unless the mothers themselves had been in accord. Women who have had one baby at home and another in the hospital almost always affirm that hospital delivery is more comfortable and more restful. But most important of all is the safety offered by hospitals in case any slight complication develops. Their laboratory equipment, their special facilities (for both mother and baby), to say nothing of the security provided by the staff of nurses and doctors, make the modern hospital the very safest place in the world to have a baby.

Rooming In: Family-Centered Care

By "rooming in" is meant a hospital program in which the infant is kept in a crib at the mother's bedside rather than in the nursery. It is an outgrowth in part of the policy of having the mother up and on her feet the day after delivery, and so taking care of the baby herself. It stems in part also from the trend toward making all phases of childbearing as "natural" as possible and fostering proper mother-child relationships at an early date. By the end of twenty-four hours the mother is generally out of bed; and thereafter, in this regimen, she conducts (under supervision by the nurses) most of the care of the infant. The mother thus becomes acquainted through actual experience with routine baby care.

Rooming in, in varying degrees, is now being used in most hospitals. In many institutions the same nurse looks after the mother and baby together. Some mothers need as much rest as possible at this time and should not be asked to shoulder the responsibilities of baby care during the first few days. Many mothers of experience hold a similar opinion, feeling that they get "rooming in" soon enough when they go home.

Alternative Birth Centers and Birthing Rooms

The hospital environment used to be a rather sterile and impersonal one for sharing the childbirth experience. Many hospitals now have birthing rooms, with a homelike atmosphere with facilities for obstetrical delivery. The labor bed also serves as the delivery table. Furnishings in the birthing room provide for the husband, and often other members of the family, to be present throughout the labor and delivery. The patient is permitted to walk and move about the room as comfort permits. Basic obstetrical supplies such as fetal stethoscope or monitoring equipment, blood pressure machines, oxygen supplies, and necessary infant resuscitation equipment are available. The room is also equipped with surgical instruments and supplies that may be required.

Some birthing rooms are right in the hospital itself and therefore offer the safety advantages of ready access to hospital specialists and equipment in the event of complications. Others are nearby in alternative birth centers and are associated with hospitals. This also provides the backup care if acute problems arise during labor and delivery.

Studies have shown that approximately 15 percent of patients in alternative birth centers, even though they enter as low-risk patients, will need acute care in modern delivery facilities. Sometimes an emergency cesarean section or an emergency vaginal operative delivery becomes necessary in the interests of either the mother or baby, or both. In obstetrical practice, these sudden emergencies frequently arise. Other times the labor may be excessively prolonged, needing a cesarean section or special method of delivery that cannot be accomplished in an alternative center.

The alternative birth centers that are located some distance from an acute-care obstetrical unit thus pose some hazards to the mother and the baby as transport systems may not be fast enough to meet sudden needs. Also, it is important for the center to have preapproved arrangements with a back-up hospital for unanticipated complications, rather than depending upon the nearest emergency room, which is often ill-equipped to take care of obstetrical problems. As we have discussed earlier, modern obstetrical practice brings to you many technological features that cannot truly be reproduced in birth centers or alternative locations, when unforeseen problems arise during labor and delivery.

Your doctor can explain in detail the availability of such alternative centers, or hospitals with such programs can provide informational brochures if you wish to consider this service. Your doctor is in the best position to advise you in regard to these plans.

It must be emphasized that such alternative centers are intended for the care of low-risk, uncomplicated mothers and infants. It is important for you to be aware that even "low-risk" situations can become "high-risk" in a matter of minutes. Thus, usually the safest place to have your baby is in a properly equipped and staffed hospital.

Home Delivery

All of the concerns expressed above apply even more to home delivery, which many patients inquire about these days. Although home delivery has obviously been satisfactorily accomplished in many situations in the past, it must be remembered that there is a three to six times higher incidence of serious problems with the baby in home deliveries. These figures are based on numerous statistics from both here in the United States and in European countries where home deliveries are often carried out under the direct supervision of a national health (usually midwife) service and therefore should be expected to give comparable results with hospital outcome statistics. However, serious problems with the newborn cannot always be foreseen, and such complications as lack of oxygen, heart irregularities, failure to initiate breathing, and birth damage usually cannot be satisfactorily managed in the average home environment. The first few moments of the newborn's life are critical ones. All of the modern methods of resuscitation, intubation, oxygen supply, maintaining newborn body temperature (avoiding cooling), and other physiological circumstances of the beginning of independent life can be fraught with the greatest dangers. It has been rightfully observed that the passage through the birth canal may be the most hazardous trip most of us will undergo in our lifetimes. Present-day technical advances in the care of the very small newborn and the compromised newborn have led to spectacular improvement in neonatal survival. Much of the needed equipment and services to achieve these improvements cannot be made available in the home and are necessarily hospital based. We urge you to consider most seriously the possible ramifications if you are thinking of home delivery. Here again it is extremely important that you have the best attention available for your pregnancy, and such care commonly consists of a properly trained physician and his or her assistants. Therefore it is imperative that you discuss the various aspects of home delivery with your physician before you embark upon such a program.

Methods of Childbirth

The crusade against pain in childbirth has a long and interesting history. Through the years the pendulum of popular as well as medical opinion in this matter has swung back and forth. Historically, the story may be said to have started with Sir James Y. Simpson's experiments in his home in Edinburgh, Scotland, in late 1847. Over the course of several evenings, Simpson and two friends had been sampling various liquid substances by inhaling their vapors, but with no result. Finally, on November 4, they tried a sweet-smelling substance, which caused them to become silly with the first whiff, drowsy with the second, and to fall asleep on the third, for a period of two or three minutes. We mention the date because it has become a landmark in the history of pain relief: these three men had just discovered the anesthetic value of chloroform.

Simpson's chief purpose in seeking a new anesthetic was to relieve the pain of childbirth. However, he faced an uphill battle to have his discovery accepted, by the public, the clergy, and the medical profession. "It is unnatural thus to interfere with the pains of childbirth, which are a *natural* function," they said. "But is not walking also a natural function?" replied Simpson. "And who would think of never setting aside or superseding this natural function? If you were traveling from Philadelphia to Baltimore, would you insist on walking the distance on foot simply because walking is man's natural method of locomotion?" Exclaimed one woman to him, "How unnatural it is for you doctors in Edinburgh to take away the pains of your patients when in labor." "How unnatural," he replied, "it is for you to have swum over from Ireland to Scotland against wind and tide in a steamboat." To the clergy's objection that such anesthesia was contrary to the Bible, with its doom for Eve: "In sorrow thou shalt bring forth children," he cited the "first surgical operation" and the "first anesthesia": "And the Lord God caused a deep sleep to fall upon Adam; and he slept; and He took one of his ribs, and closed up the flesh instead thereof." Countless other objections were raised, but to each he had an answer; he pointed out, moreover, that all things new are likely to arouse censure, particularly censure of a religious nature. Thus, he recalled, when vaccination against smallpox was introduced, various clergymen attacked the practice as irreligious, referring to it as a tempting of God's providence and therefore a terrible crime. He cited further the introduction of table forks. At first this innovation was regarded as a very sad and uncalled-for intrusion upon the old and established natural functions of the human fingers and a number of preachers denounced it "as an insult on Providence not to touch our meat with our fingers."

In various forms, the debate over pain relief in childbirth still continues. On the one hand, we have read that it is unnecessary for a woman to suffer the slightest discomfort in childbirth. Cases are described in which, almost with the first twinge of backache, the mother falls peaceably asleep with a pill or two and awakens to find the baby in her arms. The impression is given that the method is applicable in every case, never fails, and is completely harmless to mother and child; the inference has sometimes been that the mother who does not receive such pain relief has been shamefully neglected by a cruel doctor. In other articles we have found that the woman who accepts such medication not only misses a "soul-satisfying" experience but also compromises the safety of the baby for her own comfort and is hence a cowardly and selfish creature. There have been many altercations and divisions among leading obstetricians over "painless childbirth," and it is important for the expectant mother to be informed on this question.

Let us consider it further.

The Three Phases of Childbirth

For the purposes of the present discussion, the pain of childbirth may be divided into three phases. In the first place, there is a period of preliminary pains lasting, as a rule, several hours. These are comparatively mild and are rarely disturbing; even after the pains have become sufficiently definite to warrant going to the hospital, most women are able to carry on with reading or handwork after arriving there. These pains serve a useful purpose in warning that labor is starting (indeed, if the process of labor were completely painless, babies would be born in the most inconvenient places). There follows a second phase, of several hours duration, in which the pains are more severe; this comprises the greater part of the dilating phase, and as complete dilation is reached the pains usually reach their maximum. We shall return to this period soon. The third phase of pain is associated with the expulsion of the baby and lasts anywhere from about twenty minutes to two hours or more. Some form of anesthesia may be administered for the actual delivery of the baby. The type used will depend on the circumstances presented by the individual situation, on the common practice in the community, and on the preference of the mother and her obstetrician. One type is inhalation anesthesia (oxygen with an anesthetic gas); another is spinal, caudal, or epidural anesthesia (pages 147–148), eliminating all sensation in the pelvic region; while still another is local anesthesia (page 148). Vast experience has shown that these various forms of anesthesia can eliminate most of the pain associated with the expulsive stage. Furthermore, provided the mother is in a normal state of health and the baby has gone to full term, these measures are relatively safe for mother and child alike.

Since the preliminary pains are not severe enough to be disturbing, and since those of the expulsive stage may be easily decreased by anesthesia, the only pains which need concern us are those of the middle part of labor, the pains of dilation. It is over these that controversy often exists. Let us consider the usefulness and the drawbacks of a group of drugs that can be administered by injection, by mouth, or by inhalation, some of which alleviate pain and others of which, either alone or in combination, abolish the consciousness or memory of pain.

The "twilight sleep" introduced in Germany in the early years of this century was the forerunner of most of these anesthetic methods. In twilight sleep, morphine was combined with scopolamine, a drug that obliterates memory of what occurs during its influence, to achieve not only some pain relief but also forgetfulness (amnesia, which is Greek for "without memory"). This widely acclaimed and popular method ultimately proved to impose a slight but definite handicap on the baby's ability to breathe at birth and is no longer used, but it was of immense historical importance in focusing attention on the possibilities of amnesia in childbirth and pointing the way to some of our current and safer methods.

Barbiturates

Barbiturates, a group of sleep-producing drugs derived from barbituric acid, do not relieve pain but can help the mother sleep. These drugs exert a slightly depressing effect on the baby and are now used infrequently.

Demerol

Demerol is another drug that is frequently used to produce sedation and analgesia (relief of pain). It is a morphine derivative and is preferred by many doctors. Several other similar narcotic agents are available, such as Stadol and Nubain.

Although drugs, in moderate dosage, such as the barbiturates and Demerol, as well as inhalation anesthesia such as gas-oxygen, exert little or no effect on the normal full-term infant, they are likely to impair the outlook for a prematurely born baby because its incompletely developed respiratory and nervous systems are especially vulnerable to the depressing action of these agents. Hence, if you go into labor a month or more before your expected date of delivery, your physician may, for the sake of the baby, withhold these drugs and use some other method of pain relief.

Tranquilizers

Frequent use is made of the tranquilizer type of drug to ease the dilation pains of labor. These agents have some amnesic action and some muscle-relaxant effects, but their principal value lies in their ability to enhance the action of Demerol as well as to produce a sedative effect. In this way they permit the use of smaller doses of other drugs (with the reduction of possible ill effects on the baby) and at the same time they improve pain relief.

Conduction Anesthesia

It is one of the functions of the vertebral column or backbone — which is essentially a bony tube — to house the nerves along which impulses run back and forth between the brain and various parts of the body. A substantial portion of these nerves convey to the brain the various sensations received, such as the feeling of cold, heat, or pain. If any of these nerves is numbed by the application of an anesthetic drug, it is no longer able to convey impulses and hence no sensations are received by the brain from the part of the body supplied by the particular nerve or nerves anesthetized. This is the basis of spinal, caudal, and epidural anesthesia, since each entails introducing an anesthetic solution into an interior space of the vertebral column, where the drug bathes these nerves and temporarily deadens them. In these forms of anesthesia the patient is entirely conscious but is oblivious to pain or other sensations from the uterus or birth canal. This is called conduction anesthesia.

In spinal anesthesia the drug is introduced directly into the spinal canal in the region of the small of the back. It is employed chiefly for actual delivery but is sometimes used to cover the last few hours of labor. In caudal anesthesia the drug is introduced somewhat lower and into a bony space at the very lower end of the vertebral column. In epidural anesthesia the solution is introduced higher in the vertebral column. Although caudal and epidural anesthesia may be used mostly for delivery, it is usual, by renewing the anesthetic solution from time to time as its effects wear off, to make them "continuous" for as long as six to eight hours, sometimes longer, thereby enabling them to be used as labor analgesia.

Improvements in techniques and medications used for epidural anesthesia have made it considerably safer and more effective for control of labor pain. It is suitable and effective in most cases. However, if it is used too early it may slow labor and used late in labor may weaken the mother's ability to push.

Local Anesthesia

By injection of a solution containing an appropriate anesthetic drug into the tissues surrounding the vagina, the nerves that supply that area are blocked and the entire region is made insensitive to pain. Because of its high degree of safety this method has gained wide popularity for delivery. Local anesthesia of the perineal area, to permit episiotomy and expulsion of the baby, can be carried out by injecting anesthetic agents into this area. Depending upon the nerves anesthetized, these techniques are called pudendal or perineal blocks. They are especially used with the Lamaze and similar methods of childbirth (discussed below). When properly administered, local anesthetic agents have no effect on the baby, although in some cases there is a temporary slowing of the fetal heart rate.

Natural Childbirth

In recent times there has been increased interest in various forms of natural childbirth developed in the 1930s by British obstetrician Grantly Dick-Read and publicized in his book *Childbirth Without Fear*. It was his contention that fear of the anticipated pain of labor and delivery created body and muscle tensions that made the process more difficult and therefore fulfilled the fearful anticipation.

To contend with this cycle he proposed certain attitudinal approaches and training procedures as the basis of preparation for childbirth. Essential in the training procedures were proper emotional preparation, with the development of a positive attitude and understanding of the roles of medical personnel and of the birth process, and education in techniques such as proper breathing and relaxation and stretching exercises to reduce the impact of pain. While childbirth without sedation or painkillers was considered preferable, Dr. Dick-Read viewed the use of these medications as permissible where helpful or needed.

The Lamaze Method   A French obstetrician who traveled to Russia to observe procedures there, Dr. Fernand Lamaze first propounded his method in the late 1950s. The Lamaze method expands upon Grantly Dick-Read's techniques to incorporate the husband or father, or a close friend if the former are not available, as coach. The father is a participant in the classes and labor and delivery and the family unit is thereby stressed. The father works with the mother on relaxation exercises, times and literally coaches her on panting during contractions in labor, and can provide stroking or massage to ease discomfort and help distract attention from pain.

The Leboyer Technique Frederick Leboyer, another French physician, focused attention in the mid-1970s on the birth experience for the child. Feeling that the process of childbirth was a traumatic experience for the child, he suggested modifications to ease the trauma. Delivery is carried out in a quiet and preferably moderately or dimly lit room. Immediately upon the baby's emergence, he or she is placed on the mother's abdomen and cutting of the umbilical cord is delayed briefly to allow time for bonding between mother and child. Shortly thereafter the baby is given a warm, gentle bath, which can be done by the father.

Leboyer felt that easing the trauma of birth and providing opportunity for bonding would produce children who would develop into emotionally healthier adults. While there is little evidence of long-term benefits of this technique, it might enhance the experience for the participants.

The Harris and Bradley Methods The Harris and Bradley methods of "natural childbirth" are essentially modifications of the Lamaze procedure. The Harris method permits the administering of low-dose analgesics when found necessary, with an explanation of the use of such medication in labor and delivery. It is intended to eliminate feelings of "failure" some mothers experience at not coping with the pain of labor and delivery.

The Bradley method emphasizes "husband-coached" techniques in labor and delivery and the involvement of the husband in the care of the newborn. All such methods emphasize the psychoprophylactic method of understanding labor and adapting to the process by psychosomatic training and preparation.

These types of programs, many of which are rooted in principles that have been the basis of good obstetrical practice for years, are available in most areas of the country, with training classes led by qualified instructors and physicians who are familiar with the techniques. You should discuss with your doctor the pros and cons of these various methods. Remember, also, that even the most enthusiastic adherents of natural childbirth do not claim that it yields painless labor, a point that is often misunderstood. Nor does it necessarily mean drugless labor, since medication is used in many cases, although in lower dosage than would otherwise have been employed.

Since any of the drugs or methods of anesthesia mentioned above may be used either alone or in combination with any of the others listed, it is apparent that various regimens are available for the relief of pain in labor. Now, whenever many different remedies are in use for the treatment of a given condition, the chances are that no single one is entirely satisfactory. And this is very true of these drugs employed in childbirth. None is without its drawbacks; none is applicable in all cases; and none is without some slight risk to the mother or child under some circumstances. Moreoever, with a few exceptions, none can be employed except in hospitals with skilled personnel in constant attendance. It is for these several reasons that the decision in regard to the type of pain relief must rest primarily with the doctor, who is in the best position to know when these agents are safe in the individual circumstances and when they are not. Statistics show clearly that when good medical judgment is exercised in their employment, these drugs yield excellent results to both mother and child.

Accordingly, the expectant mother of today may face the pains of childbirth with genuine confidence. As we have said, the most severe pains, those of the expulsive stage, can almost always be eliminated by some form of anesthesia, while the dilation period can usually be managed in one of the ways described above. If the pains begin to be too severe for you to manage, you should so inform your doctor, who in all probability will be able to lessen their intensity at once, and certainly will do what is in the best interests of both you and your baby.

Some women request that they receive no medication for pain in labor, and most doctors are happy to comply and to give all encouragement possible. However, a do-or-die determination to go through labor without pain relief is by no means necessarily the best approach for you or the baby, and if you have made such a decision you should feel equally free subsequently to change your mind. Provided your doctor thinks that medication is appropriate, there is no more sense or glory in persisting in rejecting it than there would be for refusing anesthesia for a tooth extraction.

As we have said before, labor is undoubtedly easier for the woman who is worry-free and relaxed; in fact, the achievement of this state is itself the major factor in your being able to make the most of the birth experience and to cope with its difficulties. There are three ways to achieve it.

The transcendent prerequisite is that you have confidence not only in yourself but also in your doctor — confidence that the doctor is a medically wise, expert friend and colleague who will do everything possible for your welfare and that of your child, including working with you toward the mitigation of pain in your labor.

The second prerequisite is to acquaint yourself with the natural physiological changes that will take place in your body as pregnancy advances, so that you will know what to expect. Learn also what will happen in labor, including what the doctors and nurses will do, so that nothing will be new, unexpected, or strange. It is the purpose of this book to provide such information.

The third prerequisite is to learn to relax, a matter in which much interest has developed in recent years and which is of central importance in childbirth. Your doctor can inform you about reading material or clinics or classes that can help you to develop the capacity to relax as well as the all-important capacity to remember in labor what you have learned in practice.

11

THE BIRTH OF THE BABY

During the last few weeks of pregnancy a number of changes indicate that the coming of the infant is not far off. In a woman having her first baby, the uterus sinks downward and forward, which relieves abdominal pressure and makes breathing easier. This alteration has been called "dropping," and may occur at any time during the last four weeks, but occasionally does not happen until labor has actually begun. This sinking of the uterus is the result of the passage of the baby's head into the pelvic cavity, and in a sense is the first step in the expulsion of the child. Dropping ("lightening") often occurs suddenly, so that the expectant mother arises one morning entirely relieved of the abdominal tightness and pressure she has previously experienced. But the relief in one direction is often followed by signs of greater pressure below, particularly shooting pains down the legs, pressure on the bladder with frequent urination, and an increase in the amount of vaginal discharge. In women who have previously had children, dropping occasionally takes place during the last week or ten days of pregnancy, but is more likely to occur after labor begins.

How to Tell When Labor Begins

The onset of labor is heralded by one or more of three signs:
1. Painful, recurrent contractions of the uterus (labor pains).
2. Passage of a small amount of blood-tinged mucus ("show"), which may occur two to three days before labor.
3. Passage, usually a gush, of water from the vagina (rupture of the bag of waters, or membranes).

Contractions of the uterus occur from time to time throughout pregnancy, as evidenced by the fact that the organ now and then assumes a woody hardness. These contractions, however, are painless and occur irregularly. True labor pains are quite different from these and may usually be identified by several characteristics. In the first place, they are painful. At the onset of labor the pain is usually located in the small of the back, but after a few hours it tends to radiate girdlewise to the front. As a rule the pain begins as a slight twinge of backache, increases to a peak that is maintained a few seconds, and then diminishes gradually; in the opinion of many women it is not unlike a severe menstrual cramp. The duration of such a contraction, as well as its intensity, varies according to the stage of labor; at the outset it may not last longer than thirty seconds; later its length may range between a minute and a minute and a half. A particularly important characteristic of true labor pains is their rhythmicity. Even at the beginning of labor they are spaced at fairly regular intervals of fifteen to twenty minutes, the intervening periods being entirely free from pain. As labor progresses the pains become closer together, and within a few hours the interval is usually in the neighborhood of five minutes. Since any muscle becomes hard when it contracts, labor pains are always associated with a hardness of the uterus. This change may be readily felt by placing the hand on the abdomen during a pain.

In some instances the expectant mother has pains that seem to fill all the criteria of true labor pains but that, instead of becoming harder and more frequent, diminish in intensity after a few hours and finally disappear altogether. These "false pains" are a nuisance, since they are often difficult to distinguish from true labor. Indeed, maternity departments all over the country are continually admitting women who are apparently in labor but who report after a while that their pains have entirely stopped. The expectant mother then returns home, and though days or even weeks may elapse before effectual labor sets in, she may on the other hand be rushed back to the hospital that very night in real labor. These false alarms are a frequent source of disappointment and even of chagrin to the expectant mother, but they must be faced calmly, since there is little to be done about them. In general, false pains are characterized by the fact that their intensity remains stationary from the outset and shows no tendency to increase with time, while the severity of true labor pains increases from hour to hour; false pains, moreover, usually occur at irregular intervals in contrast to the clocklike rhythmicity of real labor; false labor pains are rarely intensified by walking about and may even be relieved, whereas true labor pains are ordinarily aggravated by the mother's being on her feet. While usually these distinguishing features are valid, there are so many exceptions that the patient must not attempt to make the differentiation herself but should notify her physician at once. If any type of painful uterine contraction is associated with a discharge of bloody mucus or of water from the vagina, it is almost certain that real labor is setting in or about to set in.

For the majority of women, labor starts by intermittent, painful contractions of the uterus, but not infrequently this is preceded (and often accompanied) by the discharge of a slight amount of blood-tinged mucus. During pregnancy the neck of the uterus is closed with a thick plug of mucus. Since, as we shall see, the process of labor entails the dilation of this canal, this plug is usually loosened and dislodged at the onset of labor and escapes through the vagina together with a drop or two of bright red blood. This phenomenon is often referred to as "show." Almost without exception, labor pains ensue within forty-eight to seventy-two hours after the appearance of "show."

Occasionally labor is initiated by rupture of the bag of waters. This may be evidenced by a sudden gush of water from the vagina or only by a slow leakage. Although this event is often followed by labor pains within a few hours, do not wait for labor pains to call the doctor, who will want to know at once if the membranes have ruptured. In the event the bag of waters should break when you are away from home, it is wise to proceed directly to the hospital, asking one of the hospital nurses or doctors to notify your medical attendant. Your suitcase can be brought later. These instructions, although they may suggest that rupture of the membranes is a serious occurrence, are given simply for the purpose of getting you to bed as soon as conveniently possible. Rupture of the bag of waters is not usually a serious event, and a vast number of perfectly normal and "easy" labors start in this manner.

Although it is commonly thought that most labors start at night, statistics show that the times of onset, as well as the times of actual birth, are rather evenly distributed around the clock. For instance, the late Dr. Joseph B. De Lee reported that in a thousand deliveries at the Chicago Lying-in Hospital, labor began and ended as follows:

Labor began		*Labor ended*
274	Between 6 P.M. and midnight	229
306	Between midnight and 6 A.M.	278
238	Between 6 A.M. and noon	267
182	Between noon and 6 P.M.	226

Accordingly, while there seems to be a slightly greater likelihood of labor's starting and ending at night rather than in the day, the tendency is not striking. It may be well to note, however, that the chances of labor's *either* starting *or* ending at night are excellent.

When to Call the Doctor

In general, the doctor should be notified as soon as you think you are in labor, as indicated by the signs just reviewed. If this is the first baby, an hour or so of regularly recurrent pains, five to ten minutes apart, that tend to increase in severity, is usually sufficient evidence. Women who have previously had children and who are therefore better able to recognize and evaluate labor pains may find it desirable to call in less than an hour, depending upon the severity of the pains, their frequency, and the patient's experience in previous deliveries. As we have already indicated, any type of painful uterine contraction when associated with "show" is strong evidence that labor is starting, and, as just emphasized, rupture of the membranes, with or without pains, demands immediate notification of the doctor. If in doubt, err on the side of calling the doctor and ask his advice.

"Overdue" Babies

As we have previously stated (page 27), the likelihood that you will start in labor on the exact day calculated for your delivery is small; the chances are one in ten, let us remember, that you will go two weeks beyond that date. This is always a trying irksome period, beset by "false alarms" no doubt, and by various discomforts — to say nothing of daily calls from solicitous friends and relatives inquiring whether pregnancy is to be your chronic state. As a result, not a few expectant mothers become impatient and want something done to initiate labor. Unfortunately, such a step is not always in the best interests of yourself and the baby, and in the long run it is usually wiser to exhaust your patience still further and wait. Very few babies are actually "overdue"; they just seem to be because unwarranted reliance has been put on the calculated date, which, as we have shown, is merely a rough estimate.

Now and then, however, there are circumstances in which your doctor, after weighing all aspects of the case, may be concerned that you are truly late, or "post-date," that is, have gone beyond forty-two weeks of gestation. There are other circumstances in which the actual "due date" cannot be determined. In such situations, the doctor may recommend various tests to assess the continued welfare of your baby. These are usually tests utilizing the elec-

The Birth of the Baby

tronic fetal monitor (p. 164), such as a test known as the non-stress test. This is done by attaching the monitoring device to your abdomen and measuring the baby's heartbeat when the baby moves about. The heart rate of the baby, like that of an adult, increases with activity.

A modification of this test is the contraction stress test, in which a variation in the baby's heart rate in response to a uterine contraction is evaluated.

These tests are harmless to you and your baby, and give valuable information regarding the baby's condition and how the baby will respond to the labor process (p. 51).

After evaluating all findings, your doctor may sometimes recommend that labor be induced. Common methods of inducing labor are injections of oxytocin (a uterine stimulant) in minute doses, and artificial puncture of the bag of waters. Provided that conditions are favorable, puncture of the bag of waters is almost always followed by labor within a few hours; but it is a procedure that should be done only when your doctor has sound reasons for it.

Admission to the Hospital

Many expectant mothers and fathers have a dread of not getting to the hospital in time. Such fears are based largely on occasional news reports of babies being born in taxicabs, on the front steps of hospitals, and in other unorthodox places. It is true that this happens now and then, but the very fact that such an event is seized upon so avidly by the press is proof enough of its rarity. Provided that ordinary common sense is used in asking the doctor's

160

advice as soon as labor seems to have begun, there is no great rush about getting to the hospital, and the trip should be made leisurely. The doctor will have notified the institution and everything will be ready for you.

For many a young woman, admission to a maternity unit marks her first real acquaintance with a hospital — though like most of us she may know well some fictional and dramatic hospital settings. The immediate reaction may be one of strangeness, of loneliness and homesickness. The nurses may seem on first acquaintance to be looking at you as "just another case," which they are dealing with in a very routine or casual sort of way. But in fact, you will find, every nurse on duty is primarily concerned with the safety of you and your child, and is prepared to do anything necessary for your well-being and that of your baby. In addition to the nursing staff, hospital house officers (interns and residents) may come into your room at odd moments, ask all kinds of questions, thump your chest, listen to your heart, and order various laboratory tests. The role of these young physicians is sometimes misunderstood by patients, so a word in their support seems in order. As medical students, these doctors of medicine have conducted dozens of deliveries and assisted at scores more; they have passed examinations in obstetrics and every other branch of medicine. At the same time these young doctors are refining their skills in obstetrics, they are giving you the benefit of having two medical attendants: your own private doctor, mature in judgment and experienced; and, as an assistant, a younger hospital physician whose special skill in certain minutiae of diagnosis and treatment is invaluable. Both are essential if the very finest type of medical care is to be given.

Things to Take to the Hospital

With few exceptions, hospitals provide everything the baby will need in the hospital. A home-going outfit will be required, of course, but whether this is taken to the hospital along with your own things or brought in to you later is a matter of personal convenience. Nor will you need very much for yourself; but it is a matter of experience that a hospital stay is somewhat more comfortable if you pack in your bag, preferably a month or so before the expected day of delivery, the following articles:

Comb, brush, and hand mirror.
Toothbrush and toothpaste.
Cologne or toilet water, deodorant.
Cosmetics, face cream, hand cream — whatever such supplies you wish.
Sanitary belt. Pads are furnished by the hospital.
Gowns. Many women prefer pajama tops to gowns; they are certainly more practical during the stay in bed.
Nursing brassieres (two), if the baby is to be breast-fed; but these pose a certain problem if purchased in advance, because they may prove to be too small after the milk comes in. It is wise, therefore, to consult your doctor about them; or if you visit the hospital where you expect to deliver, ask if nursing brassieres can be fitted and purchased in the hospital. If you do buy the brassieres before your delivery, get the adjustable kind.
Bed jacket.
Robe.
Slippers.
Clock or watch.
Pen, stationery, and stamps.
A book or two.

The Birth of the Baby

Clothes for your baby on the trip home, according to the time of year (or have them brought in later).

Preliminary Preparations for Delivery

After it is definitely established that labor is under way, the nurse carries out various preliminary preparations for delivery, the exact nature of which will depend on the wishes of the doctor and the custom of the particular hospital. The nurse assists the patient to undress, helps her into a hospital gown, and sees that she is comfortable in bed. In some instances the doctor will wish an enema to be given, in others, not; in case this is administered, a bedpan may be employed.

Then, with the nurse in assistance, the doctor — possibly your own doctor, possibly the hospital physician or attendant — examines the blood pressure, heart, and chest; a check on the latter is particularly necessary in order to make sure that there is no evidence of a recent cold or bronchitis which would have a bearing on the type of anesthesia that might be used when the baby is born. The abdominal examinations carried out at this time are the same as those made during the prenatal period, and are simply a survey to make sure the baby is in good position and that its heartbeat is audible. The nurse now drapes a sheet about the legs and thighs of the patient in preparation for an internal examination that is of the utmost importance in making certain that labor is progressing normally. These internal examinations are not disturbing if the patient will relax completely, and are usually repeated from time to time during the course of labor.

Electronic Fetal Monitoring

A number of man's greatest scientific and technological achievements have been realized through the American space program. Imagine being able to monitor a person's blood pressure, pulse, and respiration — his vital signs — when he is hundreds or thousands of miles away. Yet all this became possible through the advancements in techniques of biophysical measuring and electronic telemetry. But what has this to do with your having your baby? Simply this: that some of the great advances in computer knowledge and technology, made largely to meet the need for compact, miniaturized devices for space exploration, have been modified for use in following some of life's essential functions including childbirth. So it is that your physician can now utilize miniaturized and computerized telemetry to follow the growth, development, and health of your baby while it is still in the uterus. This is known as fetal monitoring.

Fetal monitoring is used with most patients nowadays during their labor. This entails monitoring the baby's heartbeat constantly and also evaluating the forces of labor. These techniques are commonly carried out by devices attached to the mother's abdominal wall by which the infant's heartbeat can be constantly heard and recorded. This is known as external monitoring. In some cases an internal monitor may be utilized: a tiny electrode is attached to the baby's skin on the scalp to take a direct measurement of the baby's heart rather than an indirect one through the mother's abdominal wall. By following these recordings the doctors and hospital personnel can often detect effects on the infant by such circumstances as prolonged labor or interference with the umbilical cord

The Birth of the Baby

and oxygen supply. The monitor will also indicate variations in the baby's heartbeat, which are not serious but are simply caused by normal labor contractions. In addition, in some cases a tiny sample of blood can be taken from the baby's scalp while it is still in the uterus and can be measured for various biochemical abnormalities that would indicate distress on the part of the baby.

So it is, then, that when you are in the hospital there may be a machine nearby to record your baby's heartbeat not only audibly but visually, with a permanent record if needed (see Figure 8). The monitor helps your doctor to follow the course of your labor and know if it is necessary to intervene.

What Happens in Labor

Reduced to its simplest constituents, the process of labor resolves itself into the expulsion from the uterus of the products of conception: the baby, afterbirth, membranes, and fluid. As may be seen in Figure 9, the lower portion of the uterus converges into a spindle-shaped structure, the neck of the uterus (cervix). Running through the cervix is a slender canal, which serves in the nonpregnant state for the escape of menstrual blood. Since it is through this same channel that the baby must pass, it is obvious that the neck of the uterus must dilate greatly as a preliminary to the expulsion of the infant. The greater part of labor is devoted to this dilating stage, which is usually considered the first stage of labor. During this period the contractions of the uterus exert pressure on the baby and bag of waters, forcing them gradually downward and into the cervix; by

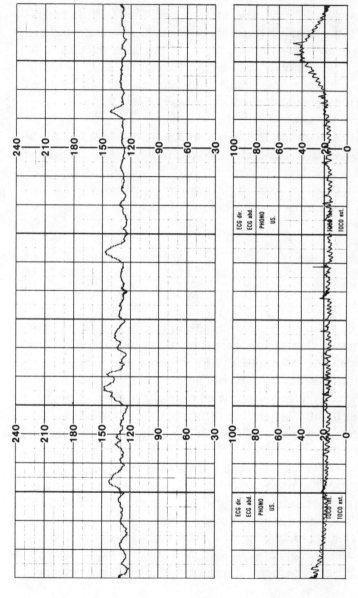

FIGURE 8. An example of a normal fetal monitoring strip. Above is the fetal heartbeat tracing, indicating normal variability measured in beats per minute, and accelerations of the fetal heartbeat. The lower tracing of uterine activity shows a uterine contraction.

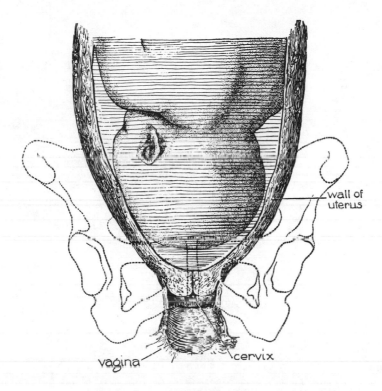

FIGURE 9. The cervix (neck of the uterus) before labor
sets in. Bag of waters intact.

this means, little by little, dilation of the canal is brought
about (Figures 9 and 10).

At the beginning of the dilating stage of labor the pains
are mild, and as we have said, occur at intervals of fifteen
or twenty minutes; but they gradually increase in severity,
and after a few hours recur every four or five minutes.

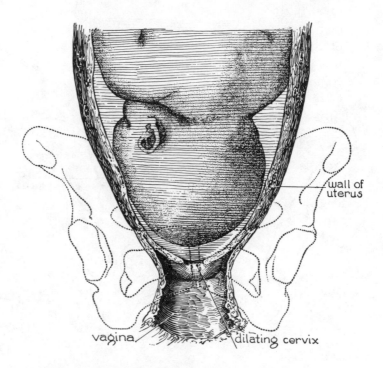

FIGURE 10. Beginning of dilation of the cervix (neck of uterus). Bag of waters still intact.

Between pains, as a rule, the patient is entirely comfortable. If the pains become exceedingly severe, it is usually possible for the doctor to administer some pain-relieving drug, a subject discussed in the last chapter (pages 144–149). During this period an effort should be made to relax as much as possible and to rest between pains; no attempt

The Birth of the Baby

should be made to "bear down" — that is, to contract the abdominal muscles in an expulsive effort such as is employed when the bowels move. This is futile at this time and merely uses up strength unnecessarily. Toward the end of the dilating stage, the bag of waters very often ruptures and the patient becomes aware of the escape of fluid. The dilation of the cervix is complete at 10 cm, or about 4 inches in diameter. Also the cervix has to efface, or thin, from about 2 cm in length to paper-thin.

The second stage of labor begins when the cervix is fully dilated (Figure 11) and ends with the birth of the child; since it is concerned with the expelling of the infant, it is often called the stage of expulsion. This stage is much shorter than the first stage, averaging something over an hour and a half with first babies and less than thirty minutes with subsequent children. It must be remembered that the expulsion of the infant is brought about by the action of the abdominal and respiratory muscles in much the same way as a bowel movement is accomplished. Accordingly, at this stage of labor, the patient may be asked to exert these muscular forces and "bear down" with each pain. A common practice is as follows: the moment the patient feels a pain coming on (there are several seconds of warning), she takes a deep breath, closes her lips, holds her breath, and strains down. Meanwhile, any local or other anesthetic has taken effect and she may carry out the desired procedure although unconscious of severe pain. With each contraction and bearing down effort of this kind, the head of the baby descends a little farther, finally distends the vaginal opening, and is born; the shoulders and remainder of the body then follow rapidly.

The degree to which the vagina is distended as the baby is born is a source of dismay to many expectant mothers,

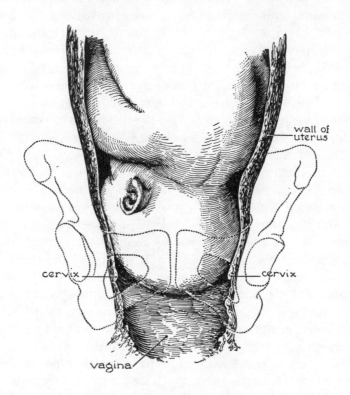

FIGURE 11. Complete dilation of the cervix (neck of uterus). The bag of waters has ruptured and the head has descended to a lower level.

who feel that deep tears must be inevitable. It is true that the vagina of the nonpregnant woman could not be stretched to any such extent. Throughout pregnancy, however, the vagina undergoes progressive changes in the way of increased succulence and distensibility, and toward the end may easily be stretched to many times its former capacity. Accordingly, the tears that do occur are usually superficial and readily repaired by a few stitches, which are taken with anesthesia. When a doctor sees that a tear is inevitable, usually a small cut is made with scissors at the place where the tear would have occurred, thus substituting for a jagged tear a straight surgical incision, which heals better; this is called an episiotomy.

The third and final stage of labor is called the placental stage, since it has to do with the expulsion of the after-birth. It rarely lasts longer than fifteen minutes and is associated with little or no pain. As a rule, the doctor assists the passage of the placenta by gentle pressure over the pubic bone. After the birth of the placenta some bleeding is normal, the quantity of blood lost averaging slightly more than half a pint. So that the bleeding does not become excessive, a uterine stimulant is frequently given and the uterus, now a hard globular mass just below the navel, may be massaged. These measures cause the interlacing muscle fibers of the uterus to contract so tightly that the blood vessels within them are squeezed shut and bleeding slows.

Duration of Labor

The length of labor varies so greatly that it is impossible to predict in a given case how long it will last. Even when labor is well under way, prophecies as to when birth will occur are of little value, since the duration of the process depends chiefly on factors that cannot be foretold; namely, the frequency and strength of the labor pains. The average duration of labor with first babies is about sixteen hours and with subsequent children eight to ten hours. The longer duration of labor in first deliveries results, of course, from the fact that the neck of the uterus, as well as the vagina, is more tense and unyielding; once these structures have been stretched by the birth of a child, they never again offer as much resistance to dilation as at the first labor. Even with a first baby, labors of less than three hours occur now and then, possibly once in a hundred cases; in later deliveries, such rapid, or "precipitate," labors are rather common, one in fifteen, perhaps. In labor exceeding twenty-four hours, the pains are usually infrequent, of short duration, and weak. In other words, here is a circumstance in which certain muscular forces have a definite task to perform; dilation of the neck of the uterus and expulsion of the baby. In some women these forces act vigorously and at frequent intervals so that the task is completed rapidly; in others they act in a more leisurely fashion and hence the process takes longer. Other things being equal, a labor of five hours and one of twenty hours may be equally normal and the outcome equally happy.

It should also be noted here that the factor of age has less bearing on the duration of labor than is generally supposed, a fact of special interest to an older woman expecting a child. The course of first labor in women over thirty-five has been the object of particular study, and the evidence is clear that there is great variety: some statistics indicate an average additional labor time of one and a half hours; others as much as four hours longer; others show a large percentage of strikingly rapid and "easy" labors in the group studied. Nor is the incidence of complications greatly higher in this older age group. Accordingly, there is no reason for the woman over thirty-five, even in her forties, to be deterred from childbirth merely by reason of

The Birth of the Baby

age. As age advances, however, the likelihood or necessity of delivery by cesarean section increases somewhat. Also, women over thirty-five have a higher risk of a child with a chromosomal (genetic) abnormality (see page 41).

Forceps Delivery

In the early decades of the seventeenth century, a new and mysterious force was making itself felt in childbirth. It became known in London that in case a woman was experiencing a prolonged labor, delivery could be effected with incredible speed if any member of a certain family of physicians was called in and allowed to take charge. The name of the family was Chamberlen. One of the Doctors Chamberlen would appear with a bundle beneath his coat and proceed to hasten delivery under cover of a large sheet or blanket so that no one could see what he was doing; a great clanking of metal would be heard and immediately the baby would be handed out from beneath the covers. Some more clanking of metal would occur and then Dr. Chamberlen, with his bundle carefully concealed under his coat, would be ready to collect his fee and depart. As a result of the metallic noises heard, and probably also because of the temporary marks that were sometimes left on the baby's head, the device by which the Doctors Chamberlen effected delivery became known as the "Hands of Iron"; and this was all that was known. For three generations — over a hundred years — this family of Chamberlens kept secret the instrument that has done more to abridge human suffering and to save human life than any other device in the whole range of surgical appliances. The "Hands of Iron," of course, were the obstetrical forceps.

173

The Birth of the Baby

The modern obstetrical forceps consist of two separate blades with smooth inner surfaces curved to fit the sides of the baby's head. After the mother has been anesthetized, the blades are inserted separately, first the left and then the right; they are next crossed and fitted together by an articulating device in such a manner that a gentle but firm grasp is obtained on the baby's head, which is then slowly extracted by means of moderate traction on the blades.

"Taking the baby with instruments" used to be regarded as an ominous procedure by the laity, and the term still has a fearsome ring to many expectant parents. Today the operation is carried out under such different conditions than formerly that it is almost a different procedure and warrants little concern. Nowadays, the majority of forceps deliveries are those in which the baby's head is almost ready to be born and are done to relieve the mother of the last fifteen or twenty minutes of labor; the head is simply "lifted out," as it were, instead of being pushed out by the expulsive efforts of the mother. It is somewhat similar to guiding the heel into a new shoe with a shoe horn. When it is best to expedite delivery in this manner depends upon the circumstances presented by the individual case, and will be determined, of course, by the medical conditions. Forceps are often used for other reasons; but the most important fact for the expectant mother and members of the family to know about these instruments is that they can be used safely only toward the end of labor, when the cervix has been fully dilated and when certain other prerequisite conditions are present. In view of this fact, the doctor should never be urged to "take the baby"; no one other than the doctor is in a position to understand whether these prerequisites have been fulfilled and to know when forceps delivery is an advantageous procedure and when it is not.

Cesarean Section

The operation of cesarean section comprises cutting through the abdominal wall and uterus and removing the child through the incisions thus made; both incisions are then carefully repaired by stitches. During recent years the incidence of cesarean section in this country has increased greatly, and today approximately ten to twenty babies in a hundred are delivered by this means. So common has the operation become that a number of women have gained the impression that this is the easiest way of having a baby and even ask the doctor if it is not possible for them to be delivered in this fashion. Such implicit faith in cesarean section is based on misinformation. Although it is true that modern surgical methods have greatly reduced the seriousness of the procedure, it is not as safe for the mother as normal delivery through the birth canal; cesarean section is a major abdominal operation, and such operative procedures are always associated with a small risk somewhat greater than that of ordinary childbirth. In well-equipped hospitals vaginal delivery can be safely carried out after cesarean section. It is, nevertheless, obligatory that every woman who has had a previous cesarean section be in the hands of an obstetrical specialist throughout any subsequent pregnancy and be delivered in a hospital.

Although cesarean section is more dangerous to the mother than *normal* childbirth, it is often safer than vaginal delivery in the presence of some types of complications.

Childbirth consists in the passage of the baby through a bony birth canal, the pelvis. Now, if the pelvis is unusually small, the baby's transit may be impeded, and under such circumstances cesarean section may be recommended by your physician. Certain other conditions also occasionally justify the use of the operation, but as we have indicated, in eighty to ninety out of a hundred cases, a mother can have her baby by the vaginal route without appreciable difficulty.

Breech Position

In about 96 percent of all cases the head of the baby is born first, but in 3 percent approximately, the buttocks of the infant enter the pelvis and, together with the legs, are the first parts to be delivered; in the latter instance the baby is said to be in "breech position." The remaining 1 percent is made up of several uncommon positions. Although a baby may be in breech position during the greater part of pregnancy, it frequently changes its position as the time of delivery approaches, the head entering the pelvis before labor starts. Breech positions carry a slightly greater risk to the infant, but in nine cases out of ten the outcome is entirely satisfactory. As far as the other is concerned, breech labor differs very little from that in which the head is born first. However, because of the risk of injury to the fetus related to breech birth, even though it is under 10 percent, many doctors will recommend cesarean section for this indication.

12

THE FIRST WEEKS
AFTER CHILDBIRTH

A period of six to eight weeks is required after childbirth for the uterus and other pelvic structures to return to their former condition. This postpartum period is referred to as the "puerperium," a term derived from the latin words *puer*, a child, and *pario*, to bear. By and large, the puerperium should be a happy and pleasant experience. As a rule, the physical discomforts are few in number and minor in character, and to offset them there is the long awaited baby, to say nothing of the fact that at last your abdomen is beginning to resume its normal proportion — which seems an almost unbelievable achievement!

At the same time, there are sound scientific grounds for believing that the nervous system or psychological state after delivery is more sensitive than at other times. Even if this were not so it would be surprising if this long-anticipated event of childbirth, with such long-term ramifications, did not evoke profound emotional responses, and occasionally troubled ones. Most common among these last is what is colloquially called the "baby blues" or "postpartum depression" that we discussed more fully back in chapter 4. As we emphasized in that discussion, the most important thing to remember is that in the great majority of cases these emotional responses are normal and not cause for great concern.

This period, from the viewpoint of mother and child alike, is of far-reaching importance, since the future health of both depends on proper rest and care during these weeks.

One of the mother's first experiences in the puerperium is the realization that the hand of a doctor or nurse is exerting pressure on her lower abdomen; actually, the hand is holding her uterus and perhaps massaging it gently from time to time. The uterus, now emptied of its contents, is the size of a large grapefruit and reaches from the pubic bone to the level of the navel. The purpose of holding or massaging it at this time is to make sure that its muscle fibers remain tightly contracted so that the amount of bleeding is minimal. Accordingly, it is customary for a doctor or nurse to place a hand on the uterus from time to time for one hour after delivery. In many hospitals this hour after delivery is spent in a recovery room. At the end of this period the mother is usually ready to return to her own room — and is also ready, as a rule, for a good rest.

During the following weeks two remarkable changes take place in the mother's body: the uterus retrogresses to its former size (involution), and milk develops in the breasts (lactation). Since most of the phenomena that occur in the puerperium are contingent upon these changes, let us consider them in some detail.

Involution of Uterus

The uterus, it will be recalled, has served a number of important purposes: it has given shelter to the infant for nine months, and through the placenta has also provided its nourishment; finally, by means of its muscular contractions, it has caused the expulsion of the baby into the outside world. Now, with its functions temporarily at an end, this structure performs the most remarkable disappearing act known to bodily economy. Within the short space of six weeks it shrinks from an organ of two pounds to one of less than two ounces. Immediately after delivery its bulk gives a distinct bulge to the lower abdomen: within a week its weight has diminished by one-half; within ten days it is usually so small that it lies entirely in the pelvic cavity and can no longer be felt through the abdominal wall. This shriveling process, by which the uterus decreases twentyfold in some six weeks, is called involution, and is brought about by shrinkage of the individual muscle cells followed by absorption of the greater part of their contents into the general circulation.

Lochia

To the mother, the most noticeable phase of involution is that in which the thickened lining of the uterus (originally prepared for the embedding of the ovum) breaks down and is cast off. This gives rise to a profuse vaginal discharge known as lochia. During the first four or five days of the puerperium this discharge contains substantial amounts of blood, mixed with cast-off cellular debris, and is consequently red in color. Toward the end of the first week the color fades to a brown; by the tenth day it has become paler, either yellow or whitish; and finally, at the end of two to three weeks, the discharge disappears almost entirely in most cases. The amount of lochia averages about one pint, three-fourths of which is discharged in the first four days; expressed in different terms, lochia requires the use of about six pads a day during the greater part of the first week. (These pads are always furnished by the hospital.) The odor of lochia resembles that of menstrual blood. After any stitches present in the perineum (episiotomy) are healed, tampons may be used. At the time of this writing, no cases of toxic shock syndrome have been reported in women in the postpartum recovery period. If tampons are used they should not be of the highly absorbent type and should be changed frequently. You should consult your doctor about resumption of use of tampons.

While the above description of lochia holds true for the average mother, great individual variation occurs in perfectly normal cases. Now and then, without apparent cause, red lochia will continue for a couple of weeks, or may reappear after several weeks on the occasion of excessive exertion. Indeed, the flow may continue off and on in small amounts for as long as four to six weeks. The Bible says "forty days." Although this prolongation of bloody lochia, or its reappearance, may be quite normal, it is often an indication that the mother is overdoing and needs more rest. If red lochia continues after four weeks, or if at any time after two weeks it is as profuse as on the first day of a menstrual period, the fact should be reported to your physician.

Lactation

In our review of the embedding of the ovum (pages 23–24), we had occasion to remark on the precision of the time relationships involved. In considering the onset of lactation, or milk secretion, we find another example of this miraculous timing. Although the breasts have been undergoing obvious preparatory changes throughout pregnancy, including the secretion of colostrum (page 5), no actual milk has been secreted, nor will any milk be secreted until after the baby is born. Regardless of whether the baby arrives a month prematurely or two weeks later than scheduled, the onset of lactation invariably occurs at the right time, namely, three days after delivery, when the baby has had time to recover from its trip through the birth canal and is ready for food. Just how nature manages this schedule is not completely known, although scientists have recently gleaned some understanding of the underlying mechanism. It now appears that hormones made by the placenta have the power of inhibiting or withholding the secretion of milk. Of course, when the baby is born, the placenta is also delivered, and when the inhibitory action of the placenta is removed, milk secretion gets under way.

Onset of Lactation

Although milk usually comes into the breasts about the third day after delivery, it is sometimes slightly later with first babies and somewhat earlier with subsequent children. The event is heralded by the breasts becoming harder, fuller, and heavier; the skin over them becomes tense, while the underlying veins become engorged with blood and appear swollen and distinct beneath the skin. If the baby is now put to the nipple a quantity of milk runs out. This fluid is quite different from the colostrum that has been secreted up to now, being of much greater volume.

The fullness of the breasts on the day the milk comes in may cause moderate discomfort, particularly in the case of first babies. This condition is not due to an inrush of milk but to the congestion in the surrounding blood vessels when the milk glands begin to function. This congestion is temporary, rarely lasts longer than forty-eight hours, and may be greatly relieved by a supportive brassiere and ice packs. Once the initial congestion is over, the breasts become softer and more comfortable.

Quantity of Milk

The quantity of milk secreted in twenty-four hours varies considerably from day to day and from mother to mother. It has been estimated, however, that the average amount secreted at first is about one-half pint daily; by the seventh day this has increased to almost a pint, while after the second week the quantity ranges from one pint to two pints or more.

A number of factors are known to affect the amount of milk a woman is able to secrete, and two of these every mother should know about. In the first place, nervous, worried, high-strung women usually have less milk than the more relaxed, serene women. Paradoxically enough, it is often the woman who is overly solicitous and concerned about having adequate milk for her baby who has the least. In other words, if you want to nurse your baby, the more you can cultivate a carefree, worry-free attitude, the most successful you will be. Second, a large intake of fluids, particularly cow's milk, unquestionably stimulates milk production. Accordingly, a concerted effort should be made to increase the amount of water and milk consumed, making sure that the total quantity of fluids taken never falls below three quarts a day. Increasing the frequency of nursing to as much as every two hours will also increase milk production, but increasing the duration of nursing each time does not seem to be effective.

Quality of Milk

Extensive investigations show that the quality of human milk varies little, provided the quantity is adequate. Nevertheless, various extraneous factors can and do affect this. For instance, almost all drugs taken by the mother reappear in the milk. In the case of cathartics this has been known since the time of the ancient Greek physicians. Alcohol passes readily into the milk, and cases are on record of babies becoming intoxicated after excessive drinking by their mothers. Nicotine appears in the milk of mothers who smoke, although the amounts are small. Again, there is a widespread belief that certain foods, such as tomatoes and pickles, affect the milk adversely and give the baby colic. Although medical opinion has long been skeptical of this fact, we are convinced, on the basis of many mothers' statements, that it contains some truth. However, we do not caution the mother against any foods, but merely suggest that if repeated trials show that certain articles of diet seem to disagree with the baby, it is only common sense to avoid them.

Time of Nursing

Most mothers are encouraged to nurse right after delivery. Usually infants require nursing about every three hours at first, although this may vary among individuals. It is customary to start with alternating breasts at each feeding, and gradually increase the duration of nursing to avoid sore nipples. Nursing can be started at five to seven minutes at first, increasing later to ten minutes or more.

Care of the Nipples

Meticulous care should be taken to keep the nipples clean. Before feedings they are usually washed with water, while between feedings it is customary for the mother to keep a pad against the nipple, being held in place by a light binder. A nursing brassiere is excellent for this purpose and is a definite help, furthermore, in preventing subsequent sagging of the breasts.

Teaching the Baby to Nurse

Although the baby is born with an active sucking reflex, many babies have difficulty in coordinating their efforts when the nipple is first put into their mouths. This sometimes seems to be the result of overenthusiasm, the baby going at the nipple with such eagerness that the nipple bobs away and the baby starts to wail. Sometimes the baby appears to become disgruntled and, after a brief trial, gives every evidence of preferring sleep to such a futile and tantalizing procedure.

Nursing is a learned skill for mother and baby. The chief purpose of putting the baby to the breast these first two days is to educate both baby and mother in the serious business of nursing. Also, the baby receives antibodies from colostrum, important in the prevention of infection. The baby should be held in such a way that the nipple can be reached with no effort whatever, no stretching of the neck to reach it, or other strain. As far as the mother's condition permits, the baby should be held in a semireclining position rather than in a horizontal one; babies take more milk in this position and are less likely to swallow air. It should also be remembered that the baby must breathe solely through the nose while suckling, and that a clear nasal pathway is essential for good nursing. If the breast is large and allowed to press against the baby's nose, it may obstruct the nasal pathway, and in the effort to breathe the baby will gulp and swallow air. Even with these precautions against swallowing air, X-ray studies show that an air bubble is almost invariably in the infant's stomach after nursing. It is therefore common practice for the mother to place the baby over her shoulder after nursing and release the bubble by gently patting the baby's back — a process referred to as "burping the baby." The hospital nurses, who will know a dozen or more tricks and maneuvers to accomplish the desired end, will be of invaluable assistance in getting suckling started. In any event, the problem involved is rarely a serious matter but merely one occasionally requiring a little patience.

Cracked Nipples

A large number of mothers have sore nipples during the early days of nursing. This condition is usually ascribable either to small cracks in the nipple or to raw areas. If nursing becomes painful, the fact should be reported to the doctor at once, for it is important that early treatment be started. Lanolin may be employed to allay the irritation (unless you are allergic to wool), and ordinarily the disturbance responds readily. Since the baby's tugging at the nipple tends to prolong the irritation, the doctor may advise a temporary decrease in the duration of nursing and the use, meanwhile, of a nipple shield or a breast pump. A nipple shield is a round glass cup that fits tightly around the outer edge of the nipple; attached to it is a rubber nipple that the child nurses. In this way the child's mouth is prevented from coming in direct contact with the nipple. A similar device is applied to the nipple when pumping is employed, artificial suction being derived either from a rubber bulb or from an electric suction apparatus. Under most circumstances the milk secured by pumping may be given to the baby in a bottle. After such measures as this have given the nipple a rest for twenty-four to forty-eight hours, direct nursing can usually be resumed without further discomfort.

Breast versus Artificial Feeding

This controversy is never offstage in discussions of the best ways to care for a baby. As was true of the controversy over pain relief in labor, the arguments on both sides of this question tend toward exaggeration. Where does the truth lie? Should you nurse your baby? Must you nurse your baby? Let us approach the question from a common-sense point of view and try to evaluate honestly the merits and drawbacks of the two methods.

The advantages of breast feeding are many:

1. Human milk is the ideal food for the newborn. It contains most of the substances necessary for maintenance, growth, and development during the first months of life in just the correct proportion for optimal digestion and absorption. Cow's milk, it must be remembered, differs from human milk in many important respects. Thus, it contains almost two and a half times as much protein as human milk; furthermore, this protein of cow's milk, when it enters the stomach, divides into relatively large curds, which are less easily digested than the fine soft curds into which the protein of human milk is dispersed. There is likewise considerable difference in the sugar content, human milk being very rich in this ingredient. Although the latter difficulty may be met by adding sugar to cow's milk, the fact remains that the *quality* of the ingredients of human milk makes it the most easily digestible

food for the newborn infant. Some infant formulas are now made that are very similar to breast milk, but they will never be identical.

2. Breast milk is normally clean; and if reasonable care is observed, the milk ingested by the baby is entirely free of harmful bacteria. Moreover, since no storing of the milk is entailed, there is no possibility of deterioration.

3. Stomach and intestinal disturbances (doubtless for the reasons just cited) are rare in breast-fed babies. Constipation is less common. In the event the stools do manifest any irregularity (change in color, consistency, etc.), there is never cause for concern since nothing can be wrong with the food and the condition is sure to right itself, whereas abnormalities of the stool in a bottle-fed baby often indicate that one or another ingredient in the formula is present in excess and a shift in the formula becomes necessary.

4. Breast milk transfers antibodies to the infant, protecting against infection.

5. Nature has packed more energy-producing value (calories) per ounce in human milk than it is usually possible to introduce into a formula. Consequently the baby receives more food as a rule, and gains more rapidly.

6. Breast feeding, through a curious connection between the uterus and breasts, hastens involution of the uterus, so that the mother's reproductive organs return to normal more rapidly.

7. Breast feeding is usually more convenient for the mother. There are no complicated formulas to measure out, no temperature levels to adjust, and no storage problems. There are no trips to the kitchen at 6 A.M. for a bottle and no standing over the stove while it warms. Breast feeding is instantly available and the simplest method of feeding the baby.

8. Breast feeding is more economical.

9. As several hundred calories per day are given to the infant in breast milk, nursing mothers find it easier to lose weight after delivery.

Expectant mothers interested in learning more about the advantages of breast feeding, or even securing personal instruction and help in the process, can contact the nearest chapter of the La Leche League. This is a nonprofit organization devoted to promoting the concepts and practice of breast feeding. If there is no local telephone listing you can write to La Leche League International, 9616 Minneapolis Avenue, Franklin Park, IL 60131 (telephone: 312-455-7730).

The merits of artificial feeding are likewise several:

1. Experience shows that mothers who rigorously follow the instructions of the doctor in the preparation of bottles and formula rarely meet difficulty in feeding their babies artificially.

2. The formula is always constant in composition and quantity; thus there is no question as to whether the milk on any particular day is adequate for the baby's needs. On the contrary, the quantity of breast milk varies not only from day to day but from feeding to feeding, being most plentiful in the morning, least in the afternoon.

3. Despite the manipulations involved in preparation of the formula, artificial feeding is less tiring to the mother and she often regains her strength more rapidly. As they say, "it takes less out of her." Moreover, the early morning bottle, or a night bottle, may be given by the husband, or other third party, while the mother sleeps.

4. If the mother is employed, artificial feeding is more convenient. However, a mother may return to work and pump her breasts at work, or nurse partially (morning and

evening). Breast milk may be stored in a refrigerator for twenty-four hours, or be frozen for the father or babysitter to use in feeding the baby.

It is barely possible that the above appraisal overstates the merits of artificial feeding, but despite this, it must be obvious that the advantages of breast feeding, as far as the baby is concerned, are considerable. As far as the health of the mother is concerned, she will probably fare as well under one regimen as under the other; as for her convenience, this will depend on individual circumstances. Returning now to our original questions, the following answers seem inescapable. Should you nurse your baby? The answer is "Yes, if at all possible." Must you nurse your baby? The answer is "No, if circumstances make it quite impossible." The woman who is able to nurse her baby should consider herself fortunate. On the other hand, the woman who is unable to do so can rest assured that artificial feeding, if meticulously carried out, will usually yield equally good results.

Health Considerations of the Puerperium

Diet
Within the first few hours following delivery, the majority of mothers are able to resume regular diet. With the birth of the baby, its demands upon the mother for nourishment do not end; they merely assume another form and continue to increase with the growth of the child. If the mother is to nurse adequately, therefore, the diet should be a generous and well-balanced one, amplified by milk or nourishing liquids between meals and at bedtime. Substantial fluid intake is important, not only because fluids

are needed in milk formation, but also because they are excreted in unusual amounts at this time in the form of perspiration. The optimal fluid intake for a nursing mother is around three quarts daily, one in the form of milk. Alcoholic drinks in small amounts (one drink) are allowed.

Bowels

Constipation is usual for two or three weeks after delivery, but as soon as normal activity is resumed the condition disappears. Your physician will order suitable stool softeners or enemas as necessary.

Bladder

The majority of women in the puerperium have no difficulty in urination, but occasionally the neck of the bladder is unavoidably compressed as the baby is born, and as a consequence the mother is unable to urinate. Sometimes very simple measures, which the nurse will suggest, suffice to relieve the difficulty, such as allowing water to run in the washbowl. If this is ineffectual, catheterization becomes necessary; that is, the urine is drained off by means of a small rubber tube inserted into the bladder. It may be necessary to repeat catheterization for a few days; if so, the procedure becomes something of a nuisance, but it is painless and need cause no concern.

Visitors

In the seventeenth century, François Mauriceau, the great Parisian obstetrician of that epoch, wrote as follows: "The Citizens Wives have a very ill Custom, which they would do well to refrain, that is, they cause their Children to be baptized the second or third Day after their labour; at which time all their Relations and Friends have a Collation in the Childbed Room, with whom she is obliged to discourse, and answer the Gossips, and all Comers a whole Afternoon together, with the usual Compliments of those Ceremonies, enough to distract her; and *tho' there is scarce any of the Company, which do not drink her Health, yet by the Noise they make in her Ears, she loses it."*

We have taken the liberty of italicizing the last lines of Mauriceau's statement, since they epitomize what happens to countless young mothers today as the result of continual salutations by well-intentioned friends. At no time is rest and quiet more needed than in the early days of the puerperium; and you yourself will realize, when the time comes, how draining it is to have to perk up and receive friend after friend (and relative after relative), all bubbling over with congratulations. During the first few days visitors should be very few — the father, parents, and possibly an intimate friend or two. While more latitude is permissible subsequently, even then it is judicious to curtail the number of visitors to two or three a day. As Mrs. Helen Washburn remarks in her delightful book *So You're Going to Have a Baby,* "You don't have to bother to explain to them about this. Nurses are expert at throwing people out."

Then, too, you must remember that nursing schedule and face the fact that your night's rest is no longer what it used to be. Accordingly a daily nap is imperative. Indeed, throughout the entire puerperium the hours between two and four in the afternoon should be reserved for you to have a complete rest.

Afterpains

Occasionally menstrual-like cramps are experienced during the first three days of the puerperium by women who have previously had children. These so-called "after-pains" are due, as a rule, to the presence of small clots in the uterus, and result from the contractions made by the uterus in its effort to expel them. The pains are likely to be particularly pronounced when the baby nurses, because of the connection that exists between the breasts and uterus (page 187). They are of no serious moment, but if they are at all severe, medication such as ibuprofen (Advil) may be helpful.

Getting Up and Going Home

As the result of shortages in hospital beds and economic pressures, it has become customary for the mother to be up earlier and thus at home sooner than formerly. Physicians and mothers everywhere have been pleasantly surprised at the results of this accelerated program — particularly with the greater rapidity with which strength is regained. Depending on circumstances, patients nowadays stay in bed only a few hours after delivery. The time of going home varies between the second and third day as a rule; the stay is usually five days after a cesarian birth.

In this connection, there is no greater boon to the young mother just home from the hospital than a mother's helper, if the baby's father or a relative or friend is not available. Such help is altogether satisfactory for this purpose, and will cost less than a nurse. Even if such an aide can be afforded for only a few days, she will be of immeasurable value to the mother during this period of readjustment. Your doctor may be able to advise you about the availability of such assistance.

It is well to recall, during these early days at home, that the pelvic organs do not return to normal until six or more weeks after delivery, and that strength returns only gradually over a corresponding interval. Do not expect to become a bundle of energy within a few short weeks. During the first two weeks at home it is best to keep stair climbing to a minimum. Mothers rarely regain their full vigor and feel their "old self" again until the baby is almost two months old.

Exercises

In order for the abdominal muscles, as well as other structures concerned in pregnancy and labor, to be restored to normal as completely and rapidly as possible, most doctors recommend an exercise program during the puerperium. Some physicians start with very simple muscular movements a day or two after delivery, while others prefer to wait until a week or ten days have passed. Since the optimal time to begin such activity depends on the circumstances of delivery and other considerations, the patient should never undertake exercising without specific instructions from her doctor. The following three exercises are particularly helpful in correcting flabbiness of the abdominal wall and in removing excess fat from the upper thighs, hips and abdomen.

1. *Leg-raising exercise* (Figure 12). Lie flat on your back with your left knee bent and raise the right foot a few inches off the bed, keeping the leg stiff; lower it slowly. Do the same with the left leg. Using each leg alternately, repeat eight times, or a fewer number if fatigued. Each day or two endeavor to raise the leg higher and higher until it is possible, without tiring, to raise each eight times to a perpendicular position. When this can be accomplished with ease, probably several weeks after delivery, raise both legs several inches off the bed (or floor), keeping the legs stiff and together. This is much more difficult and

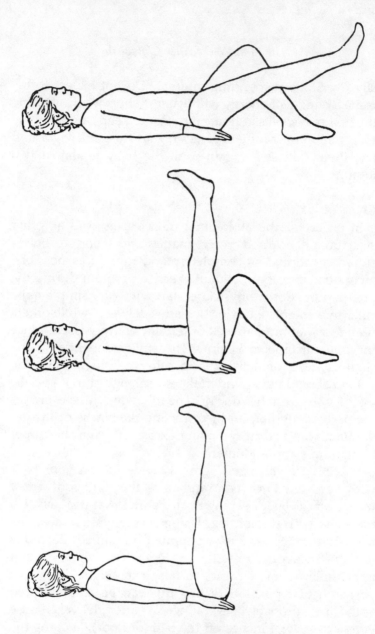

FIGURE 12. Leg-raising exercise

should not be attempted if you have back problems. Gradually, nevertheless, increase the height to which the legs are elevated until it is possible to raise both legs simultaneously to the perpendicular position. Repeat eight times.

2. *Sitting-up exercise* (Figure 13). Lie flat on your back with the arms folded across the chest and your knees bent. Raise your head off the pillow a few inches. Repeat eight times. Gradually increase the height to which the head is raised until you are able (a number of weeks after delivery) to rise to a sitting position, with the arms folded across the chest.

3. *Hip-raising exercise* (Figure 14). Lie flat on your back and raise the hips off the bed a few inches. With the hips thus elevated, contract the muscles around the rectum in the same manner in which a bowel movement is held back. Now return to the lying posture. As time goes on, increase the height to which the hips are raised and the force with which the muscles around the rectum are contracted. Do this 5–10 times at each exercise session.

With persistence, exercise of this sort will work wonders. Nothing can be accomplished in a few days, or even in a few weeks, but if the exercises are kept up for several months, those undesired pads of fat are certain to disappear.

As indicated previously, your doctor may advise variations in these particular exercises. If you have practiced yoga or similar relaxing techniques, these can be resumed as indicated by your postpartum progress.

Resumption of Tub Baths
Tub baths are permissible for the mother, as a rule, after the lochia has largely subsided. If desired, showers may be taken as soon as the mother can stand firmly on her feet, if there is a securely nonslip shower stall or bathtub.

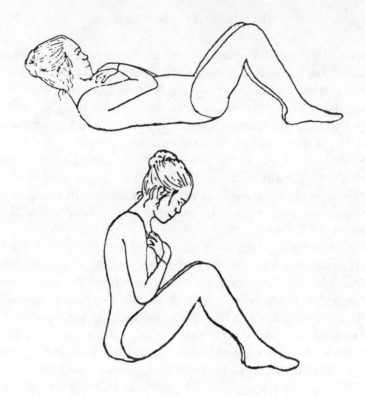

FIGURE 13. Sitting-up exercise

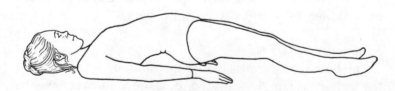

FIGURE 14. Hip-raising exercise

196

The First Weeks After Childbirth

Sexual Intercourse

It is best to defer intercourse until the lochia has ceased and any stitches (episiotomy) are well healed. It is important to remember that pregnancy might occur when intercourse is resumed, and you should consult your doctor about resumption of intercourse and birth control before leaving the hospital.

Final Examination

Some doctors make it a practice to carry out a careful pelvic examination just before the mother leaves the hospital. Almost all request that she return to the office for a final checkup when the baby is between four and six weeks old. At this time, as a rule, the mother can be assured that complete restitution of her pelvic organs has occurred and that her normal way of life may be resumed. Occasionally minor deviations from the normal are encountered, and if so, future trouble can be forestalled by suitable treatment at this time.

Return of Menstruation

In women who do not nurse their infants, menstruation usually returns within four to eight weeks after delivery, but it may not return until three to four months. Since lactation ordinarily tends to inhibit menstruation, the majority of women who nurse their babies do not menstruate for some five to six months, and not infrequently menstruation is absent as long as lactation continues. There is great individual variation, however, and sometimes a woman will menstruate despite the fact that she is nursing her baby. It should be kept in mind that although ovulation (release of the egg) does not usually take place during lactation, it still may occur occasionally and at irregular intervals. Therefore, breast feeding is no certain form of contraception, and some method of pregnancy prevention should be employed if pregnancy is not desired during this period. Combination oral contraceptive pills are to be avoided while nursing, as they may decrease the amount of milk produced. If a mother requests oral contraception during lactation, progestin-only pills are recommended. Ideally, nonhormonal methods of contraception should be utilized under these circumstances. In most mothers, the first ovulation occurs two to four weeks after cessation of lactation.

The first menstrual period after childbirth is almost always abnormal in one respect or another. It is often profuse, with clots, and may stop and later start again. This is the rule and should be of no concern. The second period is usually normal.

Activities

Your doctor will not object to your going out and driving your car, if you wish, after you have been home from the hospital a reasonable time, usually two weeks or so.

You may shampoo your hair when desired (a question often asked). Such activities as tennis, bicycling, jogging and so forth should be withheld until the lochia has ceased and the stitches are healed. More strenuous activities such as heavy lifting and heavy housework should be avoided until after your six-week checkup.

13

THE NEWBORN BABY

Although the mother often has no direct responsibility for the care of her baby during the first few hours of the puerperium, she will naturally want to acquaint herself with all that concerns this new and precious addition to the family. The baby, as soon as born, or within a few seconds, starts to cry, and generally wails lustily for a number of minutes. The abundance of air thus breathed in serves the important purpose of enriching the infant's blood with oxygen, resulting in a bright pink color. The doctor now ties and cuts the umbilical cord, and immediately the baby is launched into life as a separate individual.

Even well into the twentieth century, thousands of babies were doomed to blindness from infections (chiefly gonorrhea) contracted at birth. The great German obstetrician Karl Credé launched the virtual elimination of this cruel scourge when he discovered, in 1884, that a drop or two of a weak silver nitrate solution in each eye, dropped in immediately after birth, assured healthy eyes. This was one of the kindest contributions ever made to medicine, and gradually laws were enacted that established the now standard hospital practice of instilling a silver or penicillin preparation into the eyes of every baby shortly after birth. The antiseptic solution itself may occasionally cause mild irritation for a day or two; accordingly, if your baby develops some redness of the eyelids, along with a small amount of secretion, do not think that this is a symptom of a cold or an infection; it is merely a slight chemical irritation that is invariably harmless and of brief duration. Some hospitals are now using erythromycin ointment, as this also treats chlamydia, another cause of newborn eye inflammation, and is less likely to cause irritation.

After the eyes have been treated and a suitable dressing put on the cord, the nurse places the baby in a warm area of the delivery room and gives it its first bath. In some hospitals this takes the form of an oil bath with warm mineral oil; in others, warm water and a bland soap are used. In many hospitals no bath whatsoever is given in the belief that the vernix caseosa (page 32) is the best protective dressing that the baby's skin can have. At this time (before either mother or baby leaves the delivery room), some unmistakable identifying label is affixed to the baby; this usually consists of a string of lettered beads or a plastic I.D. band around the ankle or wrist, spelling out the mother's name. In any event, the mother may rest assured that the most meticulous labeling of each baby, before either mother or baby leaves the delivery room, is now a routine part of hospital care, and that the old fear of "mixed babies" can be dismissed. Following the bath, the baby is dressed in diapers, shirt, and gown, and placed in a warm crib.

What is it like, this new, tiny creature?

Weight

There are invariably two questions asked at once by every mother, father, and relative: Is it a boy or a girl? How much does it weigh? The former query, of course, can be answered immediately. The latter, depending on the custom of the hospital, may require an hour or two, since some institutions (and some doctors) prefer to postpone weighing the baby until it has had time to become adjusted to its new environment. If the baby is very small (premature), it may not be weighed for a day or two. Many hospitals use the metric system in weighing babies and report their weights in grams. While any doctor or nurse will be glad to convert this figure into pounds for you, you can do it yourself if you multiply the weight in grams by 22 and them mark off four decimal places from the right; in other words, multiply by .0022. For example, if the weight of the baby is 3000 grams, .0022 times 3000 equals 6.6000 pounds, that is, six and six-tenths pounds, or six pounds and approximately two-thirds. In following the weight gain of the baby from day to day — if reported in grams — it will be helpful to recall that thirty grams is about one ounce (actually, one ounce equals 28.35 grams).

Infants born at full term average about seven and one quarter pounds in weight, boys weighing usually about three ounces more than girls. Full-term newborn infants may range from five and a half pounds to eleven pounds. A weight of less than five and a half pounds ordinarily signifies that the baby has been born ahead of time and is thus a "premature" infant. However, some full-term babies may be of "low birth weight" (under five and a half pounds).

During the two days before the milk comes in, the baby undergoes a weight loss averaging about 7 percent of its birth weight; in the case of a seven-pound baby this would mean approximately one-half pound. This weight loss is due to loss of fluid and is entirely normal. Most babies make up this loss rapidly and are back at their birth weight by the tenth or twelfth day. With the exception of premature infants, babies are generally weighed daily when in the hospital. If there is any question about the amount of milk the baby is receiving, it may also be weighed before and after nursing.

Length

The average newborn baby is about twenty inches long, boys tending to be somewhat longer than girls.

Bodily Contour

A newborn infant is by no means simply the miniature of an adult, but is a creature unto itself and differs from the adult in many, many ways. Its head is proportionately large, representing about one-quarter of the body length; likewise, its abdomen is very prominent. On the other hand, the chest is narrow and the limbs are short. The legs (which in a few years will be as straight as an arrow) are so markedly bowed that the soles of the feet may nearly face each other. The neck is short because of the abundance of fat in this region. To the dismay of many parents, the baby's head is often distinctly lopsided during the first couple of weeks, and may even have a large dome-shaped lump on one side or the other. This asymmetry is due to the compression and molding the head undergoes in passing through the birth canal; it is temporary and will disappear in a week or so. Because of the large size of the head, and the weak neck muscles, the baby cannot hold its head up alone and hence the head must always be supported until the infant is about three months old. The bones making up the skull of the newborn are not joined together, but have soft membranous spaces between them. One of these spaces is quite large and may be felt as a soft, diamond-shaped depression just above the forehead. The bones surrounding this fontanel, as it is called, gradually close in, but the space is not completely obliterated until the infant is about eighteen months old.

Skin

The color of the skin varies in the newborn infant. Tiny, scarcely visible white spots are often seen on the face, particularly on the nose, but these are of no significance and disappear in a short time. The sweat glands are inactive at birth and for about a month afterward, and consequently the baby does not perspire at this period — a wise provision on the part of nature to conserve body heat and body fluids. About the second or third day the skin or eyes may assume a yellowish tinge; this jaundice of the newborn is very common and is usually regarded as a perfectly normal reaction of the baby's bodily economy to its new environment. It commonly disappears between the seventh and tenth days. Physiological jaundice of this type can be easily evaluated by measuring the bilirubin in the baby's blood. If necessary, high levels of bilirubin are often reduced by placing the baby under fluorescent lights known as bililights.

It is scarcely necessary to add that the skin of the newborn is very sensitive, and throughout the early months diaper rashes, as well as skin irritations from various causes, are common. Although these disturbances are generally minor in character, they should be reported to your physician, for early treatment usually means early cure.

Hair

The scalp at birth is covered by a variable amount of fine silky hair, usually black. About the beginning of the second week this begins to fall out and often the head is left almost bald. Gradually new hair appears, and as a rule this is firmer in texture and of different color. In other words, the appearance of the baby's hair at birth gives little clue as to what its character will be later on.

Nails

The fingernails and toenails are perfectly developed. The fingernails often extend slightly beyond the ends of the fingers, and to prevent the baby's being scratched with them, it is often necessary for the nurse to clip them early in life. As the nurse will explain to you, it is easiest to do this when the baby is asleep.

Eyes and Ears

The eyes of the newborn are peculiar in several respects. The eyebrows and eyelashes are barely discernible, being extremely short and fine. Since the tear-producing apparatus is not yet active, there are no tears at this time, no matter how hard the baby may cry, and these do not develop for several weeks; they are well established by the second month, however, and then, as if to make up for lost time — but you will find out for yourself in the due course of years. Another characteristic feature of every newborn baby's eyes is an utter lack of coordination: the eyes roll around in all directions until every new mother is certain that her child is going to be cross-eyed. Since the eye muscles have had no use in the uterus, it is understandable that they are weak at birth; with time and use they will strengthen. Light perception is present at birth, but little information can be obtained concerning actual sight. Unquestionably it becomes developed within a few days or weeks. Hearing is present even before birth, and the baby will respond to noises right away.

Breasts

Male babies as well as females often exhibit a marked swelling and hardness of the breasts during the first week, and occasionally a small amount of secretion can be expressed from the nipple. This fluid is called "witch's milk," and in medieval times was thought to have miraculous healing powers. The phenomenon is attributable to the fact that the same hormone that causes the mother's breasts to enlarge in pregnancy passes through the placenta and exerts a similar effect on the breasts of the infant in the uterus. The swelling usually subsides by the end of the first week.

Pseudo-Menstruation

"Pseudo" or false menstruation is seen in about one girl baby in twenty; it generally amounts to little more than a slight spotting of the diaper with blood for a few days. Here, again, is a condition attributable to the passage of the female hormone estrogen through the placenta, the same substance that built up the lining membrane of the mother's uterus in preparation for pregnancy (pages 23–24). All these months this substance has acted on the infant's uterus so that its lining also becomes very thick. As soon as the baby is born, this substance, which was received from the mother of course, is withdrawn and the thickened lining of the baby's uterus collapses; as a result, a slight amount of bleeding occasionally ensues.

Umbilical Cord

Since the bulk of the umbilical cord is composed of a watery, jellylike substance that surrounds the blood vessels within, the cord dries up readily when exposed to air. After the doctor cuts and ties it following delivery, a small section of an inch or so is left attached to the abdomen of the baby. As this is a potential source of introduction of infection, sometimes the cord is painted with a blue substance to prevent infection. This stump begins to shrivel the first day or two after birth, and by the end of the first week it is reduced to a small fraction of its former thickness, being little more than a dry black string. The time at which this remnant of the cord falls off varies greatly; it may separate as early as the seventh day or as late as the sixteenth or eighteenth day; the average time is around the tenth or twelfth day. This process rarely causes difficulty; when the mother leaves the hospital, the physician or nurses will give instructions about it.

Bowels

During the first two or three days the baby's stools consist of a greenish-black tarry material called meconium. This represents various products that have accumulated in the intestine before birth. After the third day the stools assume a lighter shade and are shortly golden yellow in color and pasty in consistency. During the first month of life babies have from one to four stools a day.

Circumcision

Oddly enough, the two oldest surgical operations known are both performed on the newborn infant. One of these is the cutting of the umbilical cord; the other is circumcision, or the cutting off of the foreskin of male babies. Circumcision has been carried out as a religious rite or tribal custom since prehistoric times and is still practiced, of course, by most Semitic peoples. From a medical viewpoint, there are two schools of thought in regard to this procedure. Some doctors feel that it is wise to circumcise every boy baby for purposes of cleanliness.

The American Academy of Pediatrics has recommended that circumcision is not medically necessary and need not be done routinely. Education in personal hygiene offers the same advantages as circumcision, without any risk. If circumcision is not done, it is necessary to clean under the foreskin starting at around three years of age, when the child is learning to wash himself.

Your doctor will give you advice on this question, and in case you and the father request it, will perform the operation the day before you go home or perhaps earlier. The procedure is a minor one, and when done by a doctor rarely creates the slightest disturbance. Complications have occurred, however, including infection, bleeding, and scarring.

Sleep

During the first two weeks the baby sleeps most of the time; that is, twenty to twenty-two hours a day. At this period, indeed, the baby seems to have only two interests, sleeping and eating.

Premature Infants

A baby born a month or more ahead of the expected date of delivery requires special attention. In the first place, the development of various organs is not quite complete, and accordingly the premature infant is less well equipped than the full-term one to cope with conditions outside the uterus; for instance, the lungs, nervous system, and digestive organs are weaker, and they may have difficulty in carrying out their functions. Another disadvantage is lack of fat. It will be recalled that the baby acquires most of the fat on its body during the last month in the uterus. This fat is most important in keeping the body warm, and in its absence the problem of maintaining body heat in a premature infant is sometimes most difficult. Finally, the premature baby is much more subject to infection than the full-term child.

Meticulous care makes it possible to rear an increasing number of very small babies. The prospect for infants who are very premature is dependent on the availability of neonatal intensive-care facilities. If a mother threatens to deliver prematurely, she may be transported to a hospital with an intensive-care unit for infants, as the baby will fare best if it is immediately cared for in such an environment, rather than transported after birth.

Twins

Twins occur once in eighty births approximately, triplets once in ten thousand, and quadruplets once in almost a million. More than eighty cases of quintuplets have been recorded, but with rare exceptions none of these infants has survived more than a few weeks. The first notable exception, of course, was that of the Dionne quintuplets born in Canada in 1934, and the fact that all five of these girls successfully survived infancy and childhood is one of the miracles of modern times. Recent "miracle" fertility drugs have increased the incidence of multiple pregnancies, but the hazards of prematurity yet remain.

As is well known, heredity plays an important role in twin pregnancy, and if there are already twins in the family of the expectant mother or father, the likelihood of twins is decidedly greater.

Twins are either identical or nonidentical. Identical (monozygotic) twins come from a single egg; fertilization takes place in the usual way, by a single spermatozoon, but then, very early in the egg's development, it divides into two identical parts instead of continuing as a single individual. Such twins are always of the same sex and show close physical and mental resemblances. Nonidentical (dizygotic) twins come from the fertilization of two eggs by two spermatozoa. Such twins, according to chance, may be of the same sex or of opposite sexes, and the likelihood of their resembling each other is no greater than that of any two children of the same parents. Nonidentical (or "fraternal") twins are the more common of the two types, making up about 70 percent of all twins.

It is difficult for the physician by abdominal examination of the mother to ascertain whether twins should be expected. In doubtful cases sonography may be necessary to settle the question. The latter weeks of a twin pregnancy usually are more uncomfortable for the mother than carrying a single child; heaviness of the lower abdomen, back pains, and swelling of the feet and ankles may be particularly troublesome. For this and other reasons, it is highly important for a woman with a twin pregnancy to follow her doctor's instructions with rigid care.

Twins are more likely to be born prematurely — a fact that should be taken into consideration in making plans. Many physicians will recommend bed rest from about the twentieth week, as many losses in twin pregnancies occur before thirty weeks. Even though the pregnancy goes to full term, twin babies are usually smaller than single infants by nearly a pound; however, the outlook for such babies, provided that the pregnancy continues into the last month, is almost as good as that for single infants.

Birth Certificate

Three to four weeks after delivery, you will receive by mail the baby's birth certificate. This is issued by the local health department on the basis of facts your doctor or the hospital supplies. If it has not arrived at the end of two months, inform your doctor, who will inquire into the reason for the delay.

This record is a very important document and should be carefully preserved as proof of your child's date of birth, place of birth, and parentage. It will be needed for admission to school and subsequently on many occasions (voting, passport, military obligations, and so on).

Health departments throughout the country demand that data for the birth certificate be sent to them promptly, usually within seventy-two hours after birth. This information should include the full name of the baby. If it does not, you will be asked to submit it later; but since this is something of a bother, it is desirable that you and your husband decide on a boy's name and a girl's name sometime before your expected date of delivery. To help you in reaching this decision, lists of boys' and girls' names follow this chapter.

Care of the Baby at Home

Going home with the new baby is always something of a gala occasion and it should be, for it marks the beginning of a new phase in the life of the whole family. The baby, now adjusted to conditions outside the mother's body, is ready to embark on the routine life of babyhood. The mother, in large measure restored to her previous state, is returning to her wider sphere, which now comprises many new activities involving the baby.

Prior to leaving the hospital, the mother should know how to bathe the baby, prepare its water bottle, and if a formula is used, the type of formula and how to prepare the containers. She will doubtless receive other valuable advice from the nurses about the care of the baby at home. Here, however, as in pregnancy, the mother's chief guide must be the physician. It may be that the doctor who attended you at delivery will also care for your baby at home; or, more likely, that a specialist in children (pediatrician) will be taking over. But whoever your baby doctor may be, it is highly desirable that the baby be under the doctor's surveillance during your stay in the hospital. After examining your baby carefully, the doctor will discuss with you in detail everything you need to know: food, clothes, and other aspects of the baby's care. Once this alliance is established, your child will never be farther away from the doctor than the telephone nearest you. Beyond question, such an arrangement is the surest guarantee of a healthy baby and worry-free parents.

APPENDIX I

PERSONAL NAMES

Names for Girls

Abigail: father's joy
Ada: ornament
Adela, Adelaide, Adele, Adeline: noble
Adrienne: from the city of Adria
Agatha: good
Agnes: pure
Aileen: light
Alberta: noble, shining
Alexandra, Alexis: helper
Alice, Alicia, Alison: noble
Alma: soul
Althea: healing
Amanda: lovable
Amelia, Amalia: from Roman family name Aemilius
Amy, Amata, Aimée: beloved
Andrea, Andrée: strong, brave
Angela: angel
Ann, Anna, Anne, Annette, Anita: grace
Annabel: grace, beauty
Antonia, Antoinette: priceless

April: the month April
Arabel, Arabella: merciful
Arlene: promise
Audrey: noble, strong
Augusta: royal
Ava: bird

Barbara: stranger
Beatrice: blessing
Belinda: beautiful, wise
Benita: blessed
Bernice: bringer of victory
Bertha, Berta: bright
Beryl: beryl
Beth, Betsy, Bettina, Betty (Elizabeth): God's promise
Beverly: beaver meadow
Bianca, Blanca, Blanche: white
Bonita, Bonnie: good, pretty
Brenda: sword
Bridget: strong

Camilla, Camille: temple server
Candace: pure

213

Carla, Carlotta, Carol, Carola, Carolina, Caroline: strong
Carmen: poem, song
Catherine, Catalina: pure
Cecilia: from Roman family name Caecilius
Celeste, Celia: heavenly
Charlotte: strong
Cheryl: dear
Christina, Christine: Christian
Claire, Clara, Clare, Clarice, Clarissa: bright
Claudia: from Roman family name Claudius
Clemencia, Clementine: kind
Cleo: glory
Colette (Nicole): victorious
Concepción, Concetta: beginning
Concha: shell
Constance, Constancia, Constanza: faithful
Consuela: comforter
Cora, Corinne: young girl
Cordelia: ocean gem
Cornelia: from Roman family name Cornelius
Cynthia: moon

Daphne: laurel
Deborah: bee
Della: noble
Denise: from Roman name Dionysius
Diana: light
Dinah: judgment
Dolores: grief
Donna: lady
Dora: gift
Doris: a Doric girl

Dorothy, Dorothea, Dorotea: gift of God

Eartha: earth
Edith: happiness
Edna: renewal
Edwina: happy friend
Eileen, Elaine, Eleanor, Eleanora, Elena: light
Elizabeth, Elisa, Elise, Elasabetta, Elspeth: God's promise
Ella, Ellen: light
Elma: loving
Eloise: flourishing
Elsa, Elsie: noble
Elvira: white
Emily, Emelia; see Amelia
Emma: whole
Enid: soul
Erica: queenly
Ernestine, Ernesta: earnest
Esther, Estella, Estelle: star
Ethel: noble
Eugenia: well-born
Eunice: happy victory
Eve, Eva, Evelyn: life

Faith, Fay: faith
Felicia: happy
Flora, Fleur: flower
Florence: blooming
Frances: free
Fredericka, Frieda: peace

Gail (Abigail): father's joy
Genevieve: white wave
Georgia, Georgina: farmer
Geraldine, Gertrude: spear maiden
Gladys: sword

214

Appendix I

Gloria: glory
Grace: grace
Greta, Gretchen: pearl
Guinevere, Gwendolyn: white
  wave

Hannah: grace
Harriet: queen of the home
Hazel: hazelnut tree
Helen, Helena, Helene: light
Henrietta: queen of the home
Hester: star
Hilda, Hildegarde: battle
  maiden
Holly: holly tree
Hope: hope
Hortense: gardener

Ida: happy
Imogene: image
Inez: pure
Ingrid: daughter of a hero
Iola: dawn cloud
Ione: violet
Irene: peace
Iris: rainbow
Irma: noble
Isabel: God's promise
Ivy: ivy

Jacqueline: supplanter
Jane, Janet, Janice, Jean, Jean-
  nette, Jenny: God's grace
Jennifer: white wave
Jessica: God's grace
Jewel: jewel, joy
Jill: young
Joan, Joanne, Joanna: God's
  grace
Jocelyn: just

Josephine, Josefina: increase
Joy, Joyce: joy
Juanita: God's grace
Judith: praise
Julia, Julie, Juliet: young
June: the month June
Justine: just

Karen, Kate, Katherine, Kath-
  leen, Kay: pure
Kim: ruler
Kirsten: Christian
Kit, Kitty: pure

Lana: light
Laura: laurel
Leah, Lee: weary
Leila: night
Lena, Lenore: light
Leona, Leonie: lioness
Leonora, Leonore: light
Lesley, Leslie: from surname
  Leslie
Lila: night
Lilian, Lily: lily
Linda: pretty
Lisa, Liza: God's promise
Lois: battle maiden
Lola: grief
Loretta: learned
Lorna: lost
Lorraine: from the place name
Lotta: strong
Louise, Louisa: battle maiden
Lucia, Lucille, Lucy: light
Lupe: from place name Guada-
  lupe
Lydia: from the place name
Lynn, Lynette: waterfall, lake

215

Mabel: lovable
Madeline: from Magdalene (woman from Magdala)
Madge, Maggie: pearl
Malvina: ruler
Manuela: God with us
Marcia: from Roman family name Marcius
Margaret, Margarita, Margery, Margot, Marguerite: pearl
Maria, Marie, Marian, Marianna, Marianne, Marilyn: bitter
Marjorie: pearl
Martha, Marta: lady
Mary: bitter
Mathilda, Maude: battle maiden
Maureen: bitter
Maxine: the best
May: the month May
Meg: pearl
Melissa, Millicent: bee
Mercedes, Mercy: mercy
Mildred: gentle, strong
Miranda: wonderful
Miriam: bitter
Molly: bitter
Mona: noble
Monica: adviser
Muriel: sea-bright
Myra: wonderful
Myrtle: myrtle

Nadine: hope
Nan, Nancy, Nanette: grace
Natalie: birth
Nell, Nelly: light
Nicola, Nicole, Nicky: victorious

Nina: young girl
Nita (Juanita): God's grace
Nola: bell
Nora (Honora): honor
Norma: perfect

Octavia: eighth
Olga: holy
Olive, Olivia: olive tree
Opal: opal

Pamela: honey
Patricia: noble
Paula, Pauline: small
Pearl: pearl
Peggy: pearl
Penelope, Penny: weaver
Pepita: increase
Phoebe: sun-bright
Phyllis: green branch
Polly: bitter
Priscilla: ancestral
Prudence: prudence

Rachel, Rachele, Raquel: ewe
Ramona: wise protector
Rebecca, Reba: to bind
Renata, Renée: born again
Rhoda: rose
Rita: pearl
Roberta, Robin: famous
Rona: joy
Rose, Rosa, Rosalie: rose
Rosemary: rosemary
Ruby: ruby
Ruth: beautiful friend

Sally: princess
Samantha: listener
Sandra: helper

Appendix I

Sara, Sarah, Sarita: princess
Selma: fair
Sharon: from the place name
Sheila: heavenly
Shirley: from the place name
Sophia, Sophie, Sonia: wise
Stacy (Anastasia): rebirth
Stella: star
Stephanie: crowned
Susan, Susanna, Susanne: lily
Sybil: prophetic
Sylvia: forest

Tamar, Tamara, Tammy: palm
tree
Teresa, Theresa, Terry, Tess,
Tessa: harvester
Thelma: young child
Theodora: gift of God
Tina (Christina): Christian
Toni, Tonia: priceless

Una: one
Ursula: little bear

Valerie: strong
Vanessa: butterfly
Velma: warrior
Vera: truth
Verna: flourishing
Veronica: true image
Victoria, Vicky: victory
Violet, Viola: violet
Virginia: from Roman family
name Vergilius
Vita, Vivian: life

Wanda: stem
Wendy: traveler
Wilhelmina, Willa, Wilma:
firm protector
Winifred: friend of peace

Yvonne, Yvette: yew tree

Zelda: battle maiden
Zoe: life
Zora: dawn

Names for Boys

Aaron: leader
Abel: breath
Abner: father of light
Abraham: father of multitudes
Adam: earth
Adolph, Adolfo: noble wolf
Adrian: from place name Adria
Alan, Allan, Allen: harmony
Albert, Alberto: noble, shining

Alexander, Alexis: helper
Alfred, Alfredo: wise counselor
Alphonse, Alfonso, Alonzo:
noble
Alvin: friend to all
Ambrose: immortal
Amos: burden
Andrew: strong, brave
Angelo: angel

Angus: chosen
Anthony, Anton, Antoine, Antonio, Antony: priceless
Archibald: very brave
Arnold, Arno, Arnaldo: eagle
Arthur, Arturo: noble
Augustus, Austin: royal

Barney: son of consolation
Barry: looking toward the mark
Bartholomew, Bartolomeo: farmer
Barton: barley farm
Basil: kingly
Benedict, Benito: blessed
Benjamin: son of the right hand
Bernard, Bernardo: courageous
Bertram, Bertrand: wise
Bradley: broad meadow
Brewster: brewer
Brian, Bryan: strong
Bruce: from place name Bruis
Bruno: brown-haired
Burton: fortified town
Byron: country dwelling

Calvin: bald
Cesar, Cesare: ruler
Charles, Carl, Carlo, Carlos, Carol, Carroll: strong
Chester: walled town
Christopher: Christ bearer
Clarence: famous
Clayton: clay town
Clement, Clemente: kind
Clifford: ford near a cliff
Clinton: hilltop farm
Clive: cliff

Clyde: far-sounding
Conrad: brave adviser
Cornelius: from Roman family name Cornelius
Curtis: courteous
Cyrus: sun

Dale: valley
Dana: Dane
Daniel: God is my judge
Darrell, Darryl: darling
David: beloved
Dean: official
Denis, Dennis: from Roman name Dionysius
Derek, Derrick, Dirk: ruler
Dexter: right-handed
Diego (James): supplanter
Dominic, Domingo: Sunday child
Donald: world-mighty
Douglas: dark water
Dudley: from the place name
Duncan: dark warrior
Dwight: fair

Earl: noble
Edgar: fortunate spearman
Edmund: protector of property
Edward, Eduardo: rich protector
Edwin: happy friend
Elbert: noble, shining
Eli: exalted
Eliot (Elisha): God my salvation
Elmer: noble, famous
Emanuel: God with us
Emery, Emil, Emmett: industrious

Appendix I

Enrico, Enrique: ruler of the home
Eric: kingly
Ernest, Ernesto: earnest
Ethan: strong
Eugene, Eugenio: well-born
Evan: noble young warrior
Everett: strong, brave
Ezra: helper

Felipe, Filippo: keen horseman
Ferdinand, Fernando: adventurous
Floyd: gray
Francis, Francesco, Francisco, Frank, Franklin: free
Frederick, Federico, Federigo, Fritz: peaceful king

Gabriel: strong man of God
Gary, Garrett: strong spear
Gene: well-born
Geoffrey: God's peace
George: farmer
Gerald, Gerard: strong spear
Gideon: great soldier
Gilbert, Gilberto: pledge
Glenn: valley
Godfrey: God's peace
Gordon: triangular land and hill
Graham: gray land
Grant: promise
Gregory, Gregorio: watchman
Guy, Guido: guide

Hamilton: home place
Hans (John): God's grace
Harlan, Harley: warrior
Harold, Harry: great captain

Harvey: worthy soldier
Hector: holding fast
Henry, Harry: ruler of the home
Herbert: great fighter
Herman: warrior
Hernando: adventurous
Hiram: noble
Homer: promise
Horace, Horatio: from Roman family name Horatius
Howard: protector
Hubert: bright spirit
Hugh, Hugo: brilliant
Humphrey: peace
Hyman: high

Ian (John): God's grace
Ira: vigilant
Irvin, Irving, Irwin: from surname Irving
Isaac: laughter
Ivan (John): God's grace

Jack (John): God's grace
James, Jaime, Jacob, Jacques: supplanter
Jarvis, Jervis: soldier
Jason: healer
Jasper: jasper (gem)
Jeffrey: God's peace
Jeremy, Jeremiah: exalted by God
Jerome: holy name
Jesse: God is
Joel: Jehovah is God
John, Jonathan: God's grace
Jorge: farmer
Joseph, José: increase
Joshua: the Lord is my salva-

219

tion
Juan (John): God's grace
Julio, Julian, Julius: young
Justin: just

Karl: strong
Keith: the wind
Kenneth, Kent: handsome, bright
Kermit: freeman
Kevin: handsome
Kirk: church
Kit (Christopher): Christ bearer
Knight: soldier

Lambert: light of the land
Lance (Lancelot): helper
Laurence, Lawrence, Larry, Lars: victor
Lee, Leigh: meadow
Leif: love
Leo, Leon, Leonard, Leonardo: lion
Leopold: champion of the people
Leroy: king
Lesley, Leslie: from surname Leslie
Lester: shining camp
Lewis: great warrior
Linus: flaxen-haired
Lionel: young lion
Llewellyn: ruler
Lloyd: gray
Louis: great warrior
Lucian, Lucius, Luke, Luca: light
Ludwig, Luigi, Luis, Luther: great warrior

Lyle: island man
Lyman: meadow man
Lynn: waterfall, lake

Malcolm: follower of St. Columba
Manfred: man of peace
Manuel: God with us
Mark, Marcus: warlike
Mario: masculine form of Mary
Marshall: high official
Martin: warlike
Marvin: famous friend
Mason: stonemason
Matthew: God's gift
Maurice: dark
Max, Maximilian: most excellent
Maynard: powerful
Melvin, Mervin: famous friend
Michael, Miguel: Who is like God?
Miles: strong
Milton: mill town
Morris: dark
Moses: saved from the water
Myron: fragrant

Nathan: gift
Nathaniel: gift of God
Neal, Neil: victor
Ned; *see* Edward *and* Edwin
Nelson: son of the victor
Neville, Newton: new city
Nicholas, Nick: victorious
Nils: victor
Noah: repose
Noel: Christmas
Norman, Norris: northerner

Appendix I

Ogden: valley of oaks
Olaf: ancestral
Oliver: peace
Orlando: famous
Orson: a bear
Orville: city of gold
Oscar: sacred spear
Otto: rich
Owen: noble young warrior

Patrick: noble
Paul, Pablo, Paolo: small
Percy, Percival: from surname
  Pierce
Perry: wanderer
Peter, Pedro, Pierre, Pietro: a
  rock
Philip: keen horseman
Preston: priest's town

Quentin, Quinton, Quincy:
  fifth child

Ralph, Randall, Randolph:
  counselor
Raphael, Rafael: God's healer
Raymond, Ramón: wise pro-
  tector
Reginald, Rinaldo: powerful
Reuben, Ruben: Behold, a son!
Richard, Ricardo: kingly power
Robert, Roberto, Robin: famous
Roderick, Rodrigo: famous
  ruler
Roger: wise
Roland: famous
Ronald: powerful
Roy: king
Rudolph, Rodolfo: great wolf

Rufus: redhead
Rupert: famous
Russell: redhead

Salvador: the Savior
Samuel: name of God
Sancho: holy
Saul: asked for
Scott: northerner
Seamus (James): supplanter
Sean (John): God's grace
Seth: appointed
Seymour: from place name
  Saint-Maur
Sidney: from place name Saint-
  Denis
Silas, Silvester, Sylvester: man
  of the forest
Simon, Simeon: one who hears
Sinclair: from place name
  Saint-Clair
Solomon, Sol: peace
Stanley: stony field
Stephen: crowned
Stewart, Stuart: steward

Ted; see Edward and Theodore
Terence: worn smooth
Thaddeus: praise
Theodore: gift of God
Thomas: twin
Timothy: honoring God
Tod, Todd: fox
Tony (Anthony): priceless
Tracy: path

Vaughn: small
Verne, Vernon: flourishing
Victor, Vincent, Vicente, Vit-
  torio: victor

Personal Names for Boys

Virgil: from Roman family name Vergilius
Vito: life

Wallace: Welshman
Walter: powerful ruler
Ward: watchman
Warner, Warren: defender
Wendell: rover

Wesley: west meadow
Wilbur, Willard: steadfast
William, Willis: firm protector
Wilson: son of William
Winston: firm friend
Winthrop: friendly neighbor
Woodrow: forest hedge

Zachary, Zachariah: Remember God

WEIGHTS AND MEASURES[1]

ABBREVIATIONS
For degree symbol, see Temperature, below.

C	Celsius	lb	pound
c	cup	m	meter
cc	cubic centimeter	mg	milligram
cm	centimeter	mi	mile
F	Fahrenheit	ml	milliliter
fl oz	fluid ounce	mm	millimeter
ft	foot	oz	ounce
g	gram	pt	pint
gal	gallon	qt	quart
in	inch	tbsp	tablespoon
kg	kilogram	tsp	teaspoon
km	kilometer	yd	yard
l	liter		

Weights and Measures

WEIGHT: Traditional

16 ounces = 1 pound

WEIGHT: Metric

$$\begin{array}{ccc} \mathbf{kg} & \mathbf{g}^2 & \mathbf{mg}^3 \\ 1 = 1000 & & \\ & 1 = 1000 & \end{array}$$

WEIGHT: Approximate equivalents[4]

One kilogram is approximately 2.2 pounds. To change kilograms into pounds, multiply by 2.2. To change pounds into kilograms, multiply by 0.45. In household measurements, common weights are:

```
  1 kg:   2 lb + a little more than 3 oz
500  g:   1 lb + 1½ oz
250  g:   ½ lb + 1 oz (9 oz)
100  g:   3½ oz
 30  g:   1¹⁄₁₀ oz
```

224

Appendix II

VOLUME: Traditional[5]

gal	qt	pt	cup	tbsp	tsp	fl oz
1 =	4 =	8 =	16			
	1	2	4			= 32
		1	2			16
		½	1 =	16		8
			½	8		4
			¼	4		2
				2		1
				1 =	3	½

VOLUME: Metric

The most commonly used measurements are *liter* and *milliliter*. 1 liter = 100 milliliters.[6]

VOLUME: Approximate equivalents[4]

One liter is approximately 1.06 quarts. To change liters into quarts, multiply by 1.06. To change quarts into liters, multiply by 0.95. In household measurements, common volumes are approximately:

4 l:	1 gal + 1 cup	15 ml:	1 tbsp
1 l:	1 qt + ¼ cup	5 ml:	1 tsp
500 ml:	1 pt + 2 tbsp	30 ml:	1 fl oz
250 ml:	1 cup		

LENGTH: Traditional

mile	yard	foot	inch
1 =	1760 =	5280	
	1	3 =	36
		1	12

LENGTH: Metric

km	m	cm	mm[7]
1 =	1000		
	1 =	100	
		1 =	10

LENGTH: Approximate equivalents[4]

One kilometer is approximately %10 of a mile. To change kilometers into miles, multiply by 0.6. To change miles into kilometers, multiply by 1.6.

A meter is approximately 1.1 yards (3.3 feet). To change meters into yards, multiply by 1.1; to feet, multiply by 3.3. To change yards into meters, multiply by 0.9.

Two and a half centimeters make approximately 1 inch, and 30 centimeters approximately 1 foot. To change centimeters into inches, multiply by 0.4. To change inches into centimeters, multiply by 2.5. To change feet into centimeters, multiply by 30.

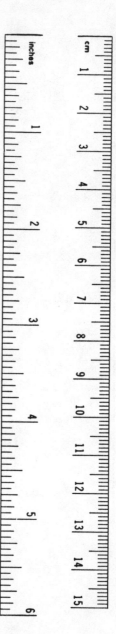

Appendix II

TEMPERATURE: Fahrenheit (traditional) and Celsius (metric)

degrees[4]

water boils at	212°F	100°C
body temperature is	98.6°F	37°C
water freezes at	32°F	0°C

To change Celsius temperature into Fahrenheit, multiply by 9/5 and then add 32. To change Fahrenheit into Celsius, subtract 32 and then multiply by 5/9.

Fahrenheit temperature

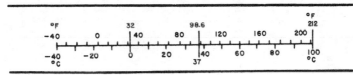

Celsius temperature

[1] Derived from material published by the U.S. Department of Commerce, National Bureau of Standards. For standard height-weight table, see page 82.

[2] A gram is a very small weight. For example, 1 tablespoon of butter or margarine weighs 14 grams.

[3] A milligram, too small for a household measure, is used in nutrition labels on packaged foods, etc.

[4] All equivalents are *approximate* except temperature, which is exact.

[5] Based on the standard 8-ounce measuring cup. All volume measurements are level.

[6] A milliliter equals a cubic centimeter, a term more generally used in medicine.

[7] A millimeter is less than one sixteenth of an inch.

FOOD ENERGY UNITS (CALORIES) IN SELECTED FOODS

(see also lists on pages 106–110)

Item and quantity	Calo-ries	Item and quantity	Calo-ries	Item and quantity	Calo-ries
MILK GROUP				(cooked)	190
				Split peas (cooked)	290
Milk (each item 1 cup)		Steak (lean and fat): sirloin	ribs 375	Lima beans (cooked;	
Whole (3.5% fat)	160	round	round 330	drained)	260
Nonfat (skim)	90		round 220		
Dry nonfat instant: 1½		Liver (fried)	195	*Nuts and peanuts* (each 1 cup)	
cups with water (1 quart)	82	Canned corned beef	185	Almonds (whole shelled)	850
Evaporated (undiluted)	345	*Lamb* (roasted; lean and fat)		Coconut (grated, firmly	
Condensed (undiluted,		Leg	235	packed)	450
sweetened)	980	Shoulder	285	Chopped walnuts	790

Food	Calories
Yoghurt (whole milk)	150
Cream (each item 1 table-spoon)	
Light (coffee)	30
Sour	25
Cheese	
Cottage (creamed): 1 cup	260
Cottage (uncreamed): 1 cup	170
Cream: 8 oz package	850
Cheddar: 1 oz	115
Parmesan (grated): 1 table-spoon	25
American: 1 oz	105

MEAT GROUP

Food	Calories
Eggs (large, 24 oz per dozen; raw or cooked in shell):	
1 egg	80
1 white	15
1 yolk	60
Meats	
Beef (cooked) (each 3 oz)	
Pot roast (lean and fat)	245
Oven roast (lean and fat):	
Pork (cooked)	
Ham (lean and fat): 3 oz	245
Bacon (crisp): 2 slices	90
Sausage	
Frankfurter (8 per pound): one	170
Salami (cooked): 1 oz	90
Poultry: Chicken (cooked)	
Broiled (flesh only): 3 oz	115
Half breast (fried)	160
Drumstick (fried)	90
Fish and shellfish	
Fish sticks (breaded, cooked, frozen): 8 oz pkg	400
Haddock (breaded, fried): 3 oz	140
Salmon (pink; canned): 3 oz.	120
Tuna (canned in oil): 3 oz	170
Clams (raw; meat only): 3 oz	65
Shrimp (canned. meat only): 3 oz	100
Dried beans and peas (each 1 cup)	
Blackeye peas (cowpeas)	245
Peanuts (roasted, salted)	840
Peanut butter: 1 tablespoon	95

VEGETABLE/FRUIT GROUP:

VEGETABLES (1 cup if no quantity given)

Food	Calories
Snap beans (cooked, drained)	30
Beets (cooked, drained, peeled, diced or sliced)	55
Beet greens (cooked, drained)	25
Broccoli (½ inch pieces) (cooked, drained)	40
Cabbage (raw, coarsely shredded)	15
Cabbage (cooked)	30
Carrots (grated raw or cooked diced)	45
Celery (raw, diced)	15
Collards (cooked)	55
Corn on the cob (5 inch ear)	70
Dandelion greens (cooked)	60
Lettuce, iceberg: 4¾ inch head	60
Onions (cooked)	60
Green peas (cooked)	60

229

Item and quantity	Calories
Green peppers (boiled):1 pod	15
Potato (boiled, 2½ inch diameter)	90
Potato (baked, 2⅓ inch diameter, 4¾ inches long)	145
Spinach (cooked)	40
Summer squash (cooked diced)	30
Winter squash (baked mashed)	130
Sweet potato (5 × 2 inches, baked in skin)	160
Sweet potatoes (canned, mashed)	140
Tomato (raw, 3 × 2 inches)	40
Tomatoes (canned, with liquid)	50
Tomato catsup (1 tablespoon)	15
Tomato juice (8 oz; 1 cup)	45
Turnips (cooked diced)	35
Turnip greens (cooked)	30

Item and quantity	Calories
Raspberries: 1 cup	70
Strawberries (capped): 1 cup	55
Watermelon: 2 pound wedge	115

GRAIN PRODUCTS

Item and quantity	Calories
Bread (18 slices per pound loaf): 1 slice Rye	60
White	70
Whole-wheat	60
Breadcrumbs (dry, grated): 1 cup	390
Cornmeal (degermed, enriched, dry): 1 cup	500
Flour (all-purpose, enriched, sifted): 1 cup	420
Flour (whole-wheat, stirred): 1 cup	400
Graham crackers (2½ inch): 2	55
Macaroni or spaghetti (enriched, cooked): 1 cup	155
Egg noodles (enriched, cooked): 1 cup	200

Item and quantity	Calories
spoon	60

MISCELLANEOUS ITEMS

Item and quantity	Calories
Baking chocolate: 1 oz	145
Semisweet chocolate pieces: ½ cup	430
Gelatin dessert powder: 3 oz package	315
Pickle (dill, 3 × 1¾ inches)	10
Tomato soup (canned, condensed, prepared with milk): 1 cup	175
Chicken noodle soup (dehydrated, dry): 2 oz package	220

VEGETABLE/FRUIT GROUP: FRUITS

Apple (2 inch diameter)	80
Avocado (10 oz)	380
Banana (medium)	100
Blueberries: 1 cup	85
Cantaloupe (half a 5 inch melon)	60
Cranberry juice cocktail (canned): 1 cup	165
Dates (dried, pitted, cut): 1 cup	490
Grapefruit half: pink	50
white	45
Lemon (2⅛ inch diameter)	20
Orange (2⅝ inch diameter)	65
Orange juice (frozen, reconstituted): 8 oz (1 cup)	120
Papaya (½ inch cubes): 1 cup	70
Peach (2 inch diameter)	35
Peaches (water pack): 1 cup	75
Pear (3 by 2½ inches)	100
Pineapple (raw, diced): 1 cup	75
Plum (2 inch diameter)	25
Prunes (dried, uncooked): 4	70

Rolled oats (cooked): 1 cup	130
Pancakes (from mix, with egg and milk): 1 cake	60
Piecrust mix (single crust): half a 10 oz package	740
Rice (white, enriched, cooked): 1 cup	225

FATS, OILS

Butter: 1 stick (½ cup)	810
Margarine: 1 stick (½ cup)	815
Vegetable fats: ½ cup	885
Salad or cooking oils (corn, cottonseed, olive, peanut, safflower, soybean): ½ cup	960
Boiled dressing: 1 tablespoon	25

SUGAR

Brown sugar, firm packed: 1 cup	820
White sugar (granulated): 1 cup	770
Table syrups (corn): 1 table-	

GOOD SOURCES OF
BASIC FOOD ELEMENTS

Most foods we eat contain a number of nutritional elements, and there are many good sources in addition to those below. Cover the four food groups every day (see summary, page 76), and vary your choice of items within each group.

PROTEIN (especially for body building, maintenance, and energy): Eggs, milk, cheese, meat, poultry, fish, dried beans and peas, whole grains and cereals, nuts. Mix animal and plant proteins at each meal for the best supply.

CARBOHYDRATES (especially for body heat and energy): Starches and sugars abound in our foods, including cakes, cookies, and so on. In choosing these generally high-calorie foods, emphasize those that supply good nutrition with the calories, such as whole-grain breads and potatoes. White sugar has 770 calories per cup.

FATS (especially for energy and some essential nutrients): Fats are enormously high in calories and so widely distributed that often too much is consumed. As with carbohydrates, look for nutrition: milk, egg yolk, nuts, peanut butter, and most cheeses give good food value. Vegetable oils (corn, cottonseed, peanut, safflower, soybean) supply essential fatty acids.

MINERALS (especially for bone structure, body functioning, red-cell formation): *Calcium:* Milk, cheese, shellfish, bone-in canned sardines and salmon, egg yolk, soybeans, green vegetables. *Iron:* Organ meats, shellfish, lean meats, soybeans and other dried beans and lentils, dried fruits, nuts, whole-grain cereals; see also the list on pages 64–66. *Iodine:* Iodized salt; seafoods. *Magnesium:* Bananas, whole-grain cereals, dried beans, milk, most dark green leafy vegetables, nuts, peanuts, peanut butter. *Phosphorus:* Whole-grain cereals, cheese, dried beans, eggs, meat, milk, peanuts, peanut butter.

Appendix IV

Other essential minerals should be supplied by a good diet with adequate protein and variety.

VITAMINS (especially for efficient use of foods in the body and maintenance of good body function): *Vitamin A:* Liver, egg yolk, deep yellow and dark green leafy vegetables (see list, pages 69–70), tomatoes, butter, margarine, whole-milk cheese. *Vitamin B₁ (thiamin):* Pork, organ meats, whole-grain breads and cereals, peas, beans, nuts, eggs. *Vitamin B₂ (riboflavin):* Organ meats, milk, cheese, meats, eggs, green leafy vegetables, whole-grain breads and cereals, dried beans. *Niacin:* Liver, meats, fish, whole-grain breads and cereals, dried peas and beans, nuts, peanut butter. *Pyridoxine (Vitamin B₆):* Bananas, whole-grain breads and cereals, chicken, dry legumes, egg yolk, most dark green leafy vegetables, most fish and shellfish, meats, liver, kidney, peanuts, walnuts, filberts, peanut butter, potatoes, sweet potatoes, prunes, raisins, yeast. *Vitamin B₁₂:* Kidney, liver, meat, milk, most cheeses, most fish, shellfish, whole egg and egg yolk. *Folacin (folic acid):* Liver, dark green vegetables, dried beans, peanuts, walnuts, filberts, lentils. *Pantothenic acid:* Organ meats, egg yolk, meats, fish, soybeans, peanuts, peanut butter, broccoli, cauliflower, sweet potatoes, peas, cabbage, potatoes, and whole-grain products. *Vitamin C (ascorbic acid):* See list, page 70. *Vitamin D:* Vitamin D milk, egg yolk, saltwater fish, liver. *Vitamin E:* Vegetable oils, margarine, salad dressing, whole-grain cereals, peanuts. *Other vitamins* are formed directly by the body, and so depend less on outside foods.

INDEX

Index

Index

Breast pump, 185–186
Breasts. *See also* Nursing
  brassieres, 86, 184
  changes, 4–5, 10, 53
  examination, 10, 37
  onset of lactation, 181–182, 197
  nipple care, 5, 87, 184–186
Breasts, baby's, 33, 205
Breathing difficulties, during
  pregnancy, 54, 118–119, 154
Breech position, 176
Burping, 185

Caffeine, 93
Calcium, 61–62, 77, 102, 232 (Appendix IV)
Calculation of birth date, 26–27, 35, 159–160
Calories (food energy units). *See also* Foods, during pregnancy; Diet; Weight, in pregnancy
  counting, 97–98
  definition, 59
  exercise and, 96
  food preparation and, 98–100
  high-calorie, low-food-value foods, 78, 97–98
  low-calorie substitutes, 78, 102
  requirements, 59
  sample menus, 106–110 (Table 2)
  selected foods and, 68–69, 104–105 (Table 1), 228–231 (Appendix III)
  2,300-calorie diet, 101–102
Carbohydrates, sources, 232 (Appendix IV)
Car seat, infant, 135–136
Castor oil, 127
Catheterization, 190
Caucasian women, and birth defects, 48–49

Caudal anesthesia, 145, 147–148
Cereals, 73–77, 103, 115, 230 (Appendix III), 233 (Appendix IV)
Cervix (neck of uterus), 130, 157, 165–170, 172 *See also* Dilation of cervix
Cesarean section, 43, 140, 173, 175–176, 192
Chamberlen family, 173
Cheeses, 63, 229 (Appendix III), 232–233 (Appendix IV)
Childbirth. *See also* Delivery; Labor
  alternative methods, 142–153
  alternative sites for, 137–142
  phases, 144–149
Childbirth Without Fear (Dick-Read), 149
Chills and fever, 84, 122, 129
Chlamydia, 200
Chloroform, 142–144
Cholesterol, 64, 66
Chorionic villus sampling, 46
Chromosomes, 21–23, 41, 43, 173
Cilia, 18
Circumcision, 207
Classes in childbirth, 40, 151, 153
Clothing
  baby, 133–134
  pregnancy, 84–86
Coffee, 93
Colace, 115
Colic, 183
Colostrum, 5, 87, 181, 184
Conception, 13, 20–21
Conduction (spinal, caudal, epidural) anesthesia, 145, 147–148
Confinement, calculating date of. *See* Birth
Constipation
  in baby, 187, 206–207

237

Index

Constipation—*(continued)*
   during pregnancy, 53, 114–116
   during puerperium, 190
Consumer Information Center, 58
Contraception, 3, 17, 197–198
Contraction stress test, 160
Contractions, 51, 88, 130, 144–
   147, 155–157, 160, 165–170
Cramps
   muscle, 84–85, 117–118
   menstrual-like, 122–123, 126,
   130, 155
Credé, Dr. Karl, 199
Curettage, 126

Danger signals, 121–131
Date of birth. *See* Birth
Datril, 94
Defects, fetal, 42–44, 46–51, 124–
   125
De Lee, Dr. Joseph B., 158
Delivery. *See also* Labor
   alternative methods, 142–153
   alternative sites, 137–142
   cesarean, 43, 140, 173, 175–176,
   192
   description, 165–171
   expected date, 26–27, 159–160
   forceps, 173–175
   preparations, 163
Demerol, 146–147
Deoxyribonucleic acid, 21
Depression, 52–53, 55–57, 177–
   178
Desserts, 78, 103
Diabetes (gestational), 47–48, 51
Diaper rash, 204
Diapers, 133–134
Diarrhea, 88, 130
Dick-Read, Dr. Grantly (*Childbirth
   Without Fear*), 149

Diet. *See also* Calories; Foods, during pregnancy; Weight, in
   pregnancy
   constipation and, 68
   deficiencies, 60
   nausea and, 111–113
   during pregnancy, 59–95
   during puerperium, 189–190
   weight control and, 95–110
   2,300-calorie, 100–101
Dieting, 60–61, 96
Dilation, of cervix, 130, 144–147,
   165–170, 172
Dionne quintuplets, 209
Discharge, vaginal
   lochia, 179–180, 195, 197–198
   nonspecific, 53, 120, 130–131,
   157
   "show," 8, 155, 157
Dizziness, 118
DNA, 21
Doctor(s)
   baby care and, 136, 211
   fee, 40
   hospital, 161, 163
   initial examination, 10–12
   miscarriage and, 124, 126
   notification of labor onset, 157–
   159
   telephoning, 130–131
   visits, 35–51, 197
Docusate, 115
Douches, 88, 120
Down syndrome, 41, 43, 47
Dried beans and peas, 64–67, 76,
   228–229 (Appendix III),
Driving, 90–91, 198
"Dropping," 154
Drugs. *See also* Anesthesia
   abortion and, 127
   abuse, 39

Index

during nursing, 183, 192, 198
during pregnancy, 78, 93–94

Echograms. *See* Ultrasound examinations

Ectopic (tubal) pregnancy, 45, 123

Egg (ovum)
  embedding, 23–24
  fertilization, 13, 20–21
  heredity, 21–23
  production, 13

Eggs, dietary, 64–67, 76, 229 (Appendix III), 232 (Appendix IV)

Eight Steps in Weight Control, 97–103

Elastic (support) stockings, 85, 117

Electronic fetal monitoring, 51, 159–160, 164–166

Embryo. *See* Egg (ovum); Fetus

Employment, 91–92, 188

Enema, 163, 190

Epidural anesthesia, 145, 147–148

Episiotomy (stitches), 148, 171, 180, 197–198

Equal, sweetener, 102

Erythromycin ointment, 200

Erythromycin, 94

Examination. *See also* Ultrasound examinations
  abdomen, 11–12, 37, 40, 163
  breasts, 10, 37
  diagnosis of pregnancy, 1–2, 10–12
  pelvis, 11, 37, 40, 163, 197
  predelivery, 163
  prenatal, 35–41
  six weeks (postpartum), 197

Exercise
  during pregnancy, 57, 88–90, 96

during puerperium, 193–195, 198

Eye blurriness, 122, 127

Eyes, baby's, 199–200, 204–205

Face, swelling of, 122, 127

Fainting, 118

Falling, during pregnancy, 85–86, 125

Fallopian tubes (oviducts), 17–21, 23

False labor, 156

Fatigue
  during pregnancy, 52, 54–55, 91–92, 125
  during puerperium, 190–191

Fats, 77, 231–232 (Appendix IV)

"Feeling life," (quickening), 7–8, 30

Feet, swelling of, 85

Fertilization (conception), 13, 20–21

Fetal alcohol syndrome, 93

Fetal monitoring, 51, 159–160, 164–166

Fetus
  defects, 42–44, 46–51, 78, 124–125
  development, 27–34, 43
  heartbeat, 7, 11–12, 30, 51, 149, 159–160, 164–166
  movements, 12, 30, 32, 51
  nourishment, 61–62
  Rh factor and, 38, 43, 48–50

Fever, 84, 122, 129

First babies, 49, 118, 154, 171–172, 181

Fish, 64, 66, 76, 78, 229 (Appendix III), 232–233 (Appendix IV)

Flatulence, 114

Fluid intake
  during nursing, 182, 189–190

Index

Fluid intake—*(continued)*
 during pregnancy, 6, 80, 113,
  115, 129
 during puerperium, 189–190
Fontanel, 203
Food, Pregnancy and Family Health
 (booklet), 58
Food elements, 59–78, 232–233
 (Appendix IV)
Foods, during pregnancy, 58–94.
 See also Calories; Diet;
 Weight, in pregnancy
 average servings, 100
 to avoid, 63, 79–80
 booklets, 58
 calorie requirements, 59, 97–98
 daily minimums 76–77
 fats and oils, 77, 231–232 (Appendix IV)
 grains group, 66, 73–77 115, 230
  (Appendix III), 232–233 (Appendix IV)
 high-calorie, 78, 97–98
 meat group, 64–67, 76, 228–229
  (Appendix III), 232–233 (Appendix IV)
 milk group, 61–64, 101–102
 preparation, 67–68, 98–100, 113
 protein requirements, 59–60, 65
 salt, 78–80, 102
 sample menus, 106–110 (Table 2)
 sugars, 79, 231 (Appendix III)
 quantity and quality, 59–61
 vegetable-fruit group, 67–73,
  76, 115, 229–231 (Appendix
  III), 232–233 (Appendix IV)
Forceps delivery, 173–175
Formula, 186–189
Fruits and vegetables, 67–73, 76,
 115, 229–231 (Appendix III),
 232–233 (Appendix IV)
Frying, 67–68, 113

Gamma globulin, 43, 50
Gas, 114
Gas-oxygen anesthesia, 145–147
Gelusil, 114
General anesthesia, 145–147
Genes, 19, 21
Genetic disorders, detection of,
 41, 43, 173
German measles, 39
Gilbert, Margaret Shea
 (Biography of the Unborn), 18
Girdles, 8, 85–86, 117
Glucose screening, 47–48
Goiter, fetal, 78
Gonorrhea, 199
Grains, 66, 73–77, 115, 230 (Ap-
 pendix III), 232–233 (Appen-
 dix IV)

Hair, baby's, 204
Hair, shampooing, 198
Hands, swelling of, 122, 127
Hands of iron, 173
Harris method of childbirth, 150
Head
 baby, 202–203
 embryo, 28
Headache, 122, 127
Health
 during pregnancy, 58–94
 during puerperium, 189–198
Heartbeat, fetal, 7, 11–12, 30, 51,
 149, 159–160, 164–166
Heartburn, 113–114
Hemorrhoids (piles), 116
Hepatitis, 39
Heredity, 16, 19, 21–23, 34–35
Hip-raising exercise, 195–196
HIV, 39
Home
 delivery, 139, 141–142
 from hospital, 192–193

Index

Index

Index

conception during, 3
menstruation and, 3
mother's attitude, 182
mother's diet, 183, 189–190
nipples, care, 184–186
time, 183–184
vs. bottle feeding, 186–189
weight of baby, 186–187
Nutrasweet, 102
Nutrition, 58–94 See also Foods
Nutritional deficiencies, 4
Nuts, 66, 76, 228–229 (Appendix III), 232–233 (Appendix IV)

Obstetrician. See Doctor(s)
Obstetric superstitions, 33–34
Oils, 77, 231–232 (Appendix IV)
Oral contraceptives, during nursing, 198
Oriental women, and birth defects, 48–49
Ovary, 13, 16–18
"Overdue" babies, 45, 51, 159–160
Oviducts. See Fallopian tubes
Ovulation
after childbirth, 197–198
periodic, 16–18
Ovum. See Egg
Oxygen-gas anesthesia, 145–147
Oxytocin, 51, 160

Pain, See also Backache; Cramps; Labor; Legs
abdominal, 122–123, 126, 130
afterpains, 191–192
during puerperium, 191–192
relief methods, 142–152, 192
round ligament, 119–120
Panty hose, 85
Pap smear, 37
Peanut butter, 66–67

Pediatrician, 136–211
Pelvis
examination, 11, 37, 85, 163
measurement, 37
Penicillin, 94
Perineal block, 148
Phosphorus, 61–63, 232 (Appendix IV)
Physician(s). See Doctor(s).
Piles (hemorrhoids), 116
Pills, contraceptive, 197–198
PKU, 102
Placenta, premature separation, 129–130
Placenta (afterbirth)
expulsion, 171
formation, 23, 25–26
role in lactation, 181
locating, 45
Placenta abruptio, 129–130
Placenta previa, 129–130
Postpartum blues, 55–56, 177–178
Postpartum period. See Puerperium
Poultry, 64–67, 76, 229 (Appendix III), 232 (Appendix IV)
Preeclampsia, 36, 39, 127–128
Pregnancy
changes during, 52–57
diagnosis, 1–2, 10–12
duration, 26
tests, 2, 37–38
ultrasound diagnosis, 2
Premature babies, 32–33, 146–147, 201–202, 208, 210
Protein
daily minimum, 64
in mother's milk, 186
intake, 59–60
sources, 62–64, 74, 101–102, 232 (Appendix IV)

243

Index

Index

Swelling
    face and fingers, 122, 127
    feet and ankles, 85
Syphilis, 38–39

Tail, of embryo, 28, 30
Tampons, 120, 180
Tay-Sachs disease, 48
Tea, 93
Teeth
    care, 87
    development in fetus, 30
Tests. See also Ultrasound exami-
    nations
    blood, 2, 37–38
    fetal monitoring, 51, 159–160,
        164–166
    pregnancy, 2, 37–38
Tetracycline, 94
Toxemia. See Preeclampsia
Toxic shock syndrome, 180
Tranquilizers, 147
Travel, 90–91, 198
Triplets, 45, 208–209
Trophoblast ("feeding" layer), 23–
    25
Tubal (ectopic) pregnancy, 45, 123
Tubes. See Fallopian tubes
"Twilight sleep," 145–146
Twins, 45, 47, 208–210
Tylenol, 94

Ultrasound examinations
    biophysical profile, 51
    course of pregnancy, 45
    diagnosis of pregnancy, 2
    fetal age, 27
    fetal heartbeat, 12, 35
    fetal position, 41
    methods, 44–45
    sex identification, 22
    twins, 209

Umbilical cord, 25–26, 164, 199
Urinalysis, 39
Urinary tract infection, 128–129
Urination
    during pregnancy, 5–6, 53
    during puerperium, 190
Urine, albumin in, 127
Urine test, for pregnancy, 2
Uterus (womb)
    abnormal shape, 125
    after birth, 171, 178, 192
    anatomy, 15–16
    contractions, 51, 88, 130, 144
        147, 155–157, 160, 165–170
    embedding of ovum in lining,
        23–24, 123
    enlargement, 8, 11
    examination, 37, 42
    formation of afterbirth, 23, 25–26
    involution, 178–179, 187
    sinking, 154

Vagina. See also Bleeding, vagi-
    nal; Discharge, vaginal
    tears, at birth, 170–171
    water discharge, 122, 130, 155,
        157
Varicose veins, 116–117
Vegetables and fruits, 67–73, 76,
    115, 229–231 (Appendix III),
    232–233 (Appendix IV)
Vegetarian alternatives, in diet,
    66–67
Venereal disease, 38–39
Vernix caseosa ("cheesy var-
    nish"), 32, 33, 200
Vision, blurred
    mother, 122, 127
    baby, 205
Visitors, after childbirth, 190–191
Vitamin A, 62–63, 66, 69–70, 76–
    77, 102, 233 (Appendix IV)

245

Index